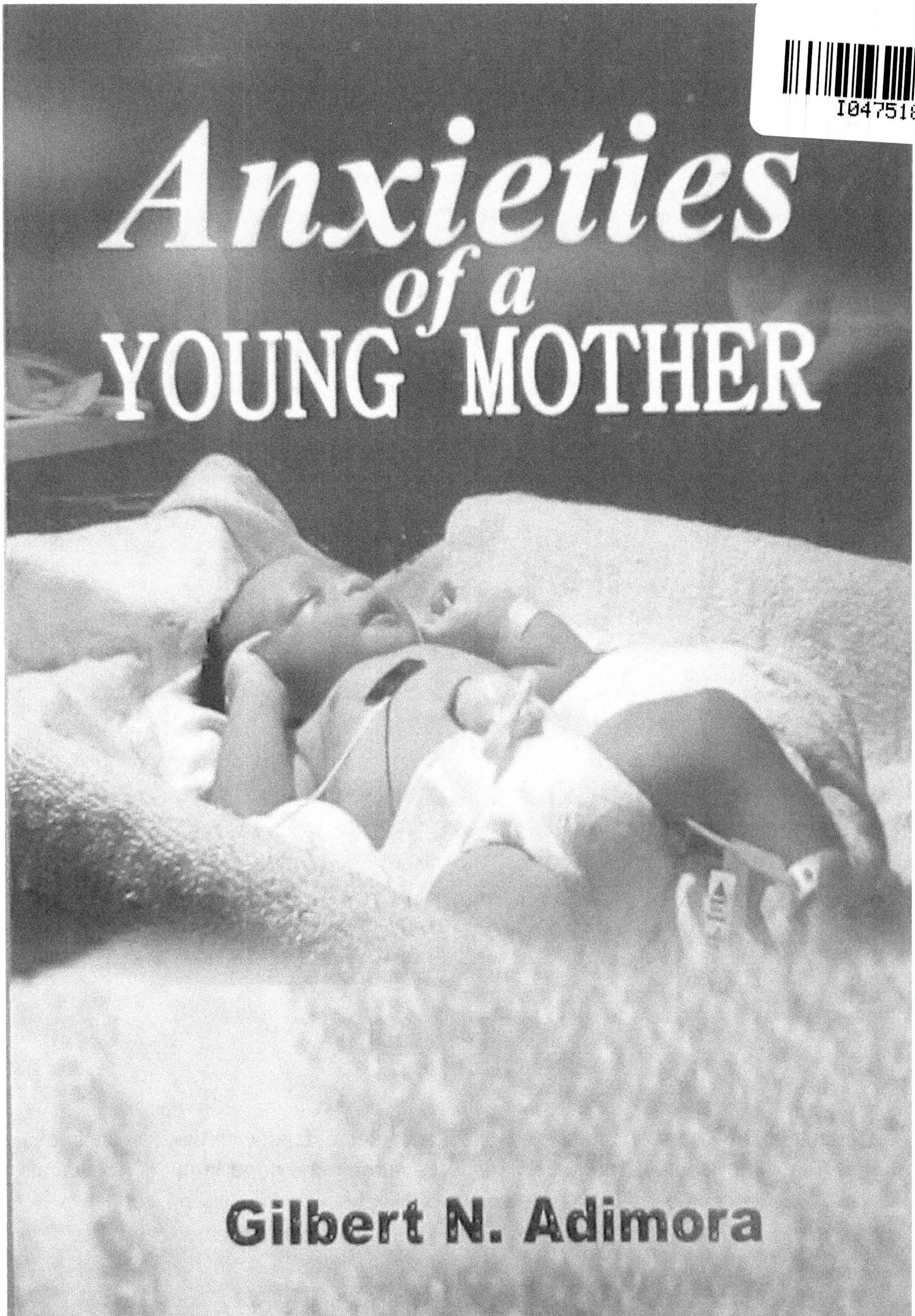

Anxieties
of a
YOUNG MOTHER

Gilbert N. Adimora

Anxieties of a young mother by Gilbert Adimora

ANXIETIES OF A YOUNG MOTHER

By Gilbert Adomora

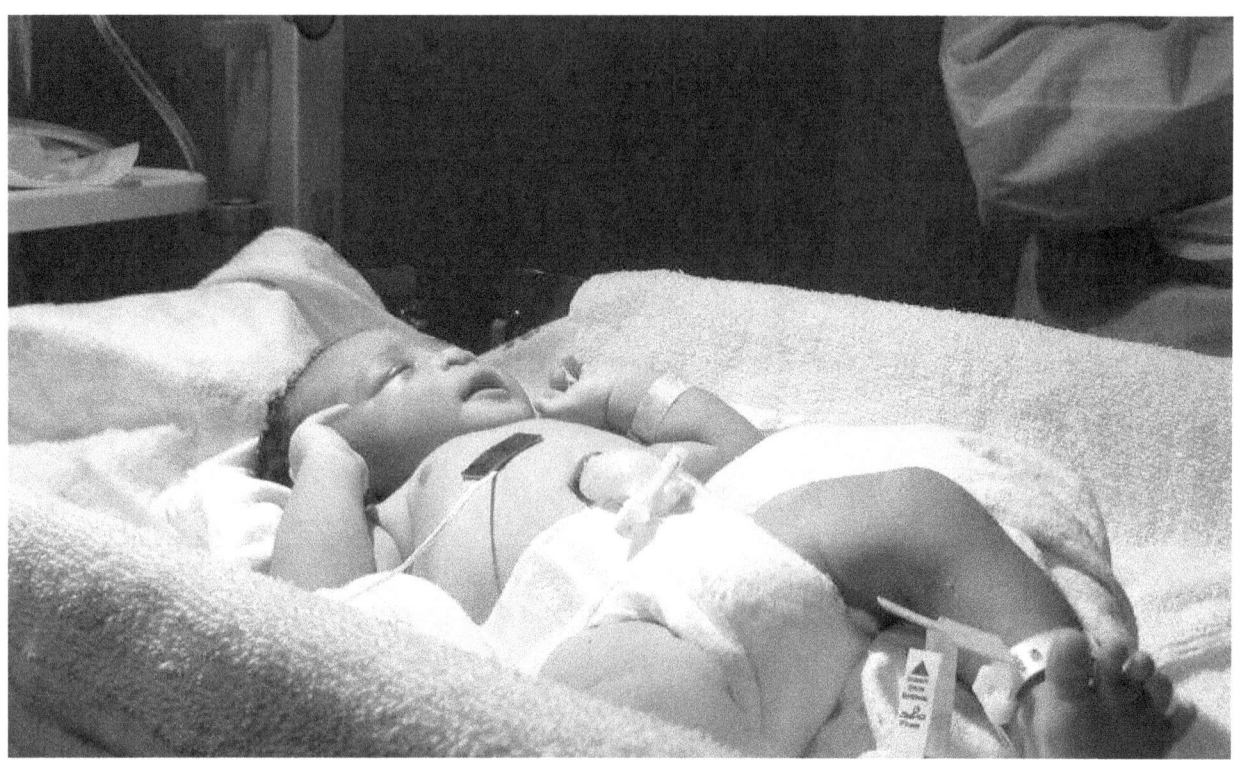

(FEATURES OFTEN SEEN IN A BABY WITHIN THE FIRST YEAR OF LIFE THAT KEEPS A MOTHER WORRIED)

The author Dr. Gilbert Adimora is a Consultant Paediatrician with the University of Nigeria Teaching Hospital, Enugu and Senior Lecturer in the department of paediatrics, college of medicine, University of Nigeria Nsukka, Nigeria.

E-mail: gilbertadimora@yahoo.com

Website: authorsden.com/gilbertadimora

Tel: 234-8033257771

Fecebook: Gilber Adimora

CONTENTS

PREFACE

This book is a written for young parents, especially those not yet experienced in the art of motherhood to help alleviate the anxieties that follow the birth and care of a new born baby till they are one year old.

Although the titleseems to focus on the mothers, fathers are not exempt and should also go through this book since they are also involved in the worry and accompanying sleepless nights.

Babies are supposed to be a desired gift from God and a bundle of joy to their parents, but often this joy is truncated by anxieties resulting from lack of knowledge, 'old wives fables', myths and cultural beliefs which are often not very accurate, sending the young parents running from place to place in search of solutions.

Funny enough, most causes of the worries are often normal processes that should take place as the newborn readjusts to life outside the mothers' womb. Some are minor problems that could be solved by a Paediatrician or good General practitioner often by counselling, bringing a much desired relief and a relaxed environment in the home.

However, a trip to the wrong place or a wrong advice from the wrong quarters could, not only permanently damage the child but also lead to the demise of the neonate or infant with much sorrow to the family.

The facts in this book are put together to help these young parents acquire the knowledge they need for the handling of their newborn babies, reduce anxiety and apply appropriate measures that will help the babies enjoy a healthy beginning in life. It is a result of many years of practice in child health both in the public and private hospital set up. It will answer a lot of questions posed by young mothers who consult paediatricians, other doctors, nurses, other health practitioners and sometimes quacks on issues that they either need not worry about or are easily sorted out by people who know what to do. It is my belief that this information will also help to reduce the incidence of ill health (morbidity) and deaths (mortality) among this age group when more parents know what to do and apply this knowledge appropriately. Mothers will also experience less anxiety especially as some mothers run high blood pressures after delivery. Any knowledge or interventions that will bring less anxiety during this period should therefore be most welcome.

1
TRANSITION BETWEEN PREGNANCY AND BIRTH.

The period between pregnancy and childbirth is usually full of anxiety, understandably so for several reasons. Labour has always been seen as a period when the life of an expectant mother hangs between life and death. However if we remember that in every situation in life we are at risk of death, many may become more relaxed and regard labour as a normal physiological process that must be experienced before a new life is brought into this planet.

In the womb, the baby's source of life (calories, proteins, fluid, oxygen and some other necessities of life) are supplied by the mother. This is through the umbilical cord which attaches the baby to the mothers' placenta on the womb through the umbilicus. The umbilicus has a network of vessels (arteries and veins) which transport these nutrients to the baby and also gets rid of the by products from the baby in the reverse direction to the mothers' system. These by products are then excreted through the mothers' various excretory system.

At the end of labour, the baby's system is detached from the mothers' and the baby now has to learn to live an independent life. A lot of readjustments have to be made to achieve this and failure in any of these leads to some of the problems experienced by some babies shortly after or sometime after birth.

Inability of the baby to breathe well (or cry) after birth may lead to lack of oxygen supply to the brain; a condition referred to as asphyxia. Asphyxia can also affect the kidneys, the heart and many other organs of the body. The duration of asphyxia in most cases determine the result or outcome of asphyxia. Permanent damage can occur in some cases especially in the brain and some people we see in the streets incapacitated especially mentally and physically may be as a result of this problem. This is referred to medically as cerebral palsy. The baby affected may not be able to sit, crawl or walk in good time leaving the parents very worried about their development. A number of them that survive become mentally handicapped and are slow in most areas of mental development. They will usually at school age need to attend special schools or care centres that are specialized in taking care of them.

Needless to say, some of these babies die during delivery because of the problems earlier mentioned.

It is very important to note that the most effective way of avoiding this problem is prevention. Mothers should attend antenatal clinics when they are pregnant so that any problems that may arise during delivery will be anticipated and steps taken to avoid them.

Many of the babies that develop asphyxia is because the baby is either too big to pass through the birth canal, or the mothers' birth canal is too narrow to allow the baby pass through making normal delivery difficult or even impossible. An operation or some other form of medical intervention is therefore needed to deliver the baby alive and well.

Unfortunately, some mothers refuse consent for an operation because of cultural reasons. It is either that other women would look at them as weaklings because they could not put to bed *normally* or that they do not want to have a scar on their abdomen. In either case, it is better to have a healthy baby than to listen to other peoples' comments or have a *clean* abdomen without a scar but a damaged baby that cannot go to school and remain an embarrassment and burden to the family for life.

The lives of the mothers are also put at a high risk when they refuse to have an operation. Many mothers have died in the process leaving their precious babies motherless. The better option is very obvious in these situations.

The other conditions that may lead to difficult deliveries include bad positioning of the baby. For instance, a baby may be lying across (transverse) in the womb instead of the head being in the pelvis as is usually the case. Some babies may have their lower limbs and buttocks in the pelvis (breech). In some cases, the head may be abnormally big, usually due to infections inside the womb affecting the brain, or malformations especially of the brain during development in the womb.

ALL these conditions can be detected by good ante natal care especially with recently introduced equipment like the *Ultrasound* and other equipment that monitor the baby and the mother before and during labour. This goes a long way to promote safe delivery of the baby and the mothers' good health.

It may also be important here to mention spiritual reasons as some of the reasons why some women do not want to have any medical intervention in form of an operation. They think it is 'exercising faith' to go into labour and deliver *'like Hebrew women'* some of them would say.(Exodus 1:19). I believe that nothing can be further from the truth. Faith is a lifestyle and should not be practiced only when we feel like avoiding a situation or when there is trouble. I also believe that our Creator is very interested in mother and baby's safety after delivery. He gave the knowledge for the developments we have in all fields of medicine to help mankind. Be sure He is supporting your faith action and that you have always been used to His voice before taking your faith decision.

Since we have earlier mentioned malformations in this discussion, it may be important to advice mothers to avoid taking medications not approved by their doctors, herbs and roots during pregnancy to avoid adverse effects on the babies. Some medications are well known for their adverse effects on the newborn babies and have been banned from distribution.Others are still in circulation because of their usefulness in other disease conditions but are not to be taken during pregnancy.

In the case of roots and herbs, it is advisable that they be avoided completely during pregnancy for the safety of the baby. This is simply because most of them have not been adequately tested to know whether they affect the baby in any way. I have personally in my practice seen two babies whose mothers admitted to taking herbs to keep the babies small so that delivery will be easier. However, both babies did not survive apparently because of their very low birth weights and possibly because of possible damage to the vital internal organs bythe herbs the mothers ingested during pregnancy. The small size of the babies could mean that some of the internal organs could also be equally too small to function effectively

Mothers should also endeavour to feed well during pregnancy; taking food that is rich in proteins, iron and vitamins. Our normal local food in Nigeria usually contains enough carbohydrates. Vitamins may be very important in the formation of tissues and organs of the unborn child. A recent survey carried out in the United States indicates that incidence of *spina bifida* (a malformation of the spine and the spinal cord which can cripple a child) can be reduced by as much as 85% if the mother of the baby takes adequate quantities of folic acid during pregnancy.[1]

2

THE FIRST DAY OF LIFE

The first day of life is full of anxieties for the young mother especially those giving birth for the first time (primips) or those who have had one or two sad experiences in the past.

BREATHING

Because the most obvious sign of life in a human being is breathing, young mothers often watch the breathing of their newborn babies very closely. Unfortunately, because the breathing pattern of the new born baby is *'not normal'* like that of adults, some mothers rush to the doctor with complaints that the baby is not breathing well.

A newborn baby sometime breathes fast, at other times he seems to 'suspend' breathing for sometime and then starts off once more. This should not be a cause for concern. It is not an indication that the baby is not well. This breathing pattern changes a few days after birth.

A common fear of the mother is whether the baby was suctioned well after delivery and that if this is not properly done the baby will develop respiratory problems. Any baby whose airways are not properly cleared may not be able to leave the delivery room because of irritation. Mothers should rest assured that so far as the baby is breathing normally, the airways are clear. However any rapid respiration especially when associated with grunting should be reported to the doctor.Noisy breathing sounds from the baby should also be reported to the doctor.

3
EARLY FEEDING

In some of our cultural beliefs babies are not supposed to be given anything except plain water in the first two days of life. This is believed to help wash the baby's stomach before real feeding can be started. This practice is dangerous especially for babies that have gone through difficult or prolonged labour. The reason is that the calories in the baby gets 'burnt out' during labour because of the intermittent contractions of the uterus and the caloric demands from the baby to meet the needs. The longer this persists, the lower the caloric stores in the body and the baby is either delivered with low caloric stores or may already have low blood sugar. Starving the baby further by giving only plain water tips the baby into low blood glucose (hypoglycaemia). This can lead to seizures (convulsions) and if not immediately controlled, can cause irreversible brain damage.

If the mother is not stable or fit after delivery, the baby can be started on artificial formula *on doctors' prescription* until the mother improves. *Exclusive breastfeeding, except where not indicated is the feeding of choice.*

Babies should be put to breast within 30minutes of delivery if the baby and the mother are stable. Contrary to the belief in some quarters, the first flow of milk from the mother after birth is NOT harmful to the baby; it is actually very beneficial to the new born baby as we are going to see in further discussion on breast feeding.

4
FIRST STOOLS

Most babies pass the first stool within the first 48 hours of birth, some may delay for up to 4 days and this should not be a cause for concern. The first stool passed (meconium) is usually dark, greenish and sometimes slimy. This should again not bother the mother because they are normal. However if a baby has not passed any stools after 3-4 days *and the abdomen is distending,* the doctor's opinion should be sought.

Lose watery stools within the first 24hours of birth,especially when passed several times in a day needs medical attention.

URINE

Some mothers observe that their babies have not made any urine within the first 24 hours because the diapers are not wet. Their worry is justified, but there are some reasons for this. The baby may not have been fed since birth and therefore hasn't much fluid to pass out. This means that the baby could actually at this point be dehydrated. All that is needed is to feed the baby properly and wait. If this is done most of them will make urine within a couple of hours after the feeding. If after feeding the baby does not still make urine, medical attention should be sought.

Coloured urine, mainly yellowish discoloration, may be seen a few days after delivery. This should not also be a cause of anxiety; however if the urine has an odour or is blood stained, proper investigations need to be carried out and treatment initiated if necessary.

A baby that cries each time he/she is passing urine also needs to be seen by the medical staff for investigation. *Please note that this is not the same as a baby that cries because the diapers are wet.* This is usually due to discomfort from the wet diapers and is normal.

5

THE EYES OF THE NEW BORN

A normal baby may not open the eyes as the mother would wishand seems to be sleeping all the time. This is normal but a careful observer will notice that the baby actually opens the eyes at intervals. Most newborn babies sleep most of the time and only wake up when they are hungry. Some mothers worry that their baby sleeps most of the time only waking up at intervals to feed. This should not be a source of anxiety since it is normal.

Eye discharge is a relatively common occurrence in newborn babies but this is dealt with in a later chapter.

Some mothers may notice a patch of redness usually on one side of the white area of the eyeball after delivery and get worried enough to rush back to the doctor for intervention. Most of the time this red patch is a very small bleed under the white of the eye (conjunctiva). It is caused by pressure on the eyes when the baby was passing through the birth canal. No treatment is needed as the redness usually clears after a few days without any intervention.

6

FEVER IN THE NEW BORN

Fever can occur in newborn babies and should be taken seriously with the understanding that early intervention, if need be will save the parents from a lot of stress and the baby unnecessary suffering. Fever can be of different types

DEHYDRATION FEVER

New born babies can develop a fever if they are not fed early after delivery. This is usually called dehydration fever since it is a response of the brain to inadequate volume of fluid in the circulation. This is common within the first two days of life. The solution is to feed the baby with breast milk if this has started running or with artificial feeds on prescription if the mother is indisposed. Drugs are not usually necessary since the fever subsides after feeding the baby. Some people give plain water for this purpose but it is better to feed the baby properly so as to provide both the calories and the required fluid at the same time.

HIGH ENVIRONMENTAL TEMPERATURES.

Sometimes when the environmental temperatures are high, babies start to run a fever because of immaturity of the area of the brain that controls body temperature. This is more common in premature babies but can occur in any newborn. It is usually observed that the fever occurs at the time of the day when temperatures are highest (Usually from 2pm to 4-5pm in Nigeria).

Exposing the baby is usually enough to bring down the temperature. Unfortunately most mothers feel that babies should be properly covered all the time no matter the temperature of the environment. Their reason is that these babies could develop 'cold in the chest' (pneumonia) if exposed. This is definitely not the case. A mother should use the way she feels to determine whether the baby will be dressed in warm clothing, light clothing or exposed fully.

INFECTIVE FEVER

If after the measures described above a baby still has persisting fever, medical attention is required. This should be done as early as possible to enable the medical team intervene and expect a better outcome of treatment. The causes of infections in babies are very many and medication at home may not be the best for newborn babies because their condition could deteriorate rapidly. In the past, new born babies hardly suffered from malaria because of the immunity acquired from their mothers. Because of the changes in the nature of the malaria parasite this is no longer so. We now see a lot of newborn babies with malaria and some of them have high fever.

Bacterial infection can also lead to high body temperatures in newborn babies. Since some of these infections are contacted while the baby is still in the womb, the infections may have been established and advanced before delivery. Parents are therefore advised not to delay before seeking medical attention.

IMMUNIZATION FEVER

Some babies may develop a fever after their first immunization which is usually BCG and OPV. The cause of the fever is usually obvious because of the timing of the fever which starts soon after immunization. More common however is fever following immunizations at 6weeks, 10weeks and 14 weeks the so called triple vaccine (against diphtheria, pertussis and tetanus). Simple analgesics like paracetamol are usually enough for treatment of the fever which usually subsides a couple of days later. If however the fever persists and is of a high grade, medical attention should be sought so that the patient can be appropriately investigated and treated.

7

THE EYES.

The eyes of a newborn baby can also be a cause of concern for the mother for many reasons. Generally babies do not open their eyes easily for one to see but when they do, a few things can be seen which can cause anxiety for the mother.

REDNESS OF THE EYES. (SUBCONJUNCTIVAL HAEMORRHAGE)

In some babies, after birth a patch of red area can be seen on the conjunctiva (the white of the eye) as if something has hit the eye. Naturally this is a cause of concern for the mother. This patch of redness is caused by pressure on the eyes when the babywas passing through the birth canal. The pressure leads to the rupture of some tiny vessels in the areas where the pressure is highest, but this is usually minimal. This condition needs no treatment as the red area disappears after some days.

However,if the eyes are uniformly red and with possible discharge of clear or coloured fluid, medical attention is needed.

EYE DISCHARGE.

A few days after birth some babies develop yellowish or whitish or watery eye discharge which in some cases may cause the eyelids to stick together especially in the mornings. Most eye discharges in babies are caused by infective organisms usually contacted through the mothers' birth canal during the process of delivery. They should be properly treated and in doing so the mother ideally should also receive treatment to avoid infecting future babies. Depending on the organism causing the infection, eye discharge in babies should be easily treated.

Some mothers are advised to use their *breast milk* to treat eye discharge as eye drops. This is not in any way helpful and could actually endanger the babies' eyes by worsening the infection. Breast milk is usually sterile but can also be contaminated and infect the baby's eyes. Apart from this it is also a good medium for growth of infective organisms which can harm the eyes.

Herbs and other remedies are not advisable for use in the treatment of eye discharges in babies especially now that effective, easy to apply drugs are available. The doctor should be consulted as early as possible.

YELLOWNESS OF THE EYES (JAUNDICE).

The most common cause is jaundice which is fully dealt with in a subsequent chapter.

SQUINT.

This is when the two eyes are not pointing in the same direction when focusing on an object as should be the case. This should not be a source of worry. The child should be handled by an ophthalmologist when he/she is a little older.

DROOPING EYELIDS (PTOSIS)

I have seen some mothers worried about this rare feature of the upper eyelids. Usually involving one upper eyelid, the affected lid droops lower than the other side. In most babies this feature runs in families and one or more older relations may be seen with the same feature. Most times nothing can be done about this, but more importantly it doesn't have any effect on the child's sight. The child can see normally. The only problem is only cosmetic. An ophthalmologist should however be consulted to carry out proper examinations to confirm that there are no other problems.

8

RECURRENT VOMITING

This condition can be very frightening and distressing to mothers. A newborn baby starts vomiting repeatedly after birth and this seems to occur with each feed. If untreated the baby gets progressively weaker because of the energy expended while vomiting and compounded by poor feeding which results in low calories available for the babies' metabolism.

One of the most common causes of this condition is the irritation of the walls of the stomach by swallowed amniotic fluid by the baby during delivery. Untreated, this may persist for several days and in some cases unnecessarily aggressive and potentially harmful remedies may be applied. The affected babies need to be treated in a hospital set up where the stomach could be washed out. As soon as this is done the baby experiences some relief and start feeding properly.

In some cases some other conditions or causes that are easily treatable may be responsible for the recurrent vomiting. Medical attention and intervention are required in this case.

9

INITIATING FEEDING

Most new born babies should be able to start breast feeding within one hour of birth. This assumes that the mother is well and stable after delivery. Ideally a new born baby should be put to the mothers' breast soon after birth. There are some advantages in this. The bond (closeness) between the mother and the baby is made stronger. Apart from this, the mothers' breast starts to run much earlier because of the stimulation from the baby's suckling.

Labour puts a baby through a lot of stress and this may make them come out with low blood sugar. This can be corrected early if the baby is fed as soon as possible after delivery.

There is a common belief that a baby should not be given anything but water at least for 2 days after delivery. The reasons are to get rid of the first flow of milk which is not good for the baby and also to allow the baby's be prepared to receive the mothers or else the baby will develop abdominal gripes (pains). Both of these beliefs are wrong. The baby's stomach, even when premature is very ready to receive milk and digest it.

   The old belief is that the mothers' first flow of breast milk is not suitable and is unsafe for the baby is wrong. In fact there are advantages in making sure that the baby gets, if possible all this first milk. It is called colostrum in medical terms and actually contains a lot of human protein products called immunoglobulin that protects the child from infective organisms. It also contains more protein and calories than the milk that flows later.

Sometimes the flow of milk starts late and is a source of concern for the parents. This may be due to the psychological state of the mother. Many mothers are psychologically stressed after during and after delivery especially during the first pregnancy. A mother who is not relaxed may not be able to produce breast milk early and in good quantity.

In some special cases doctors prescribe infant formula for feeding of the baby till the breast starts to flow. During this period it is advised that the mother should put the baby to breast before feeding with formula so that the suckling will help the breast start to produce milk early.

Any child in who breast feeding has not been established 48 hours after delivery should be taken for medical attention.

A baby on exclusive breast feeding does not need water since the breast milk contains enough water to meet the needs of the baby.

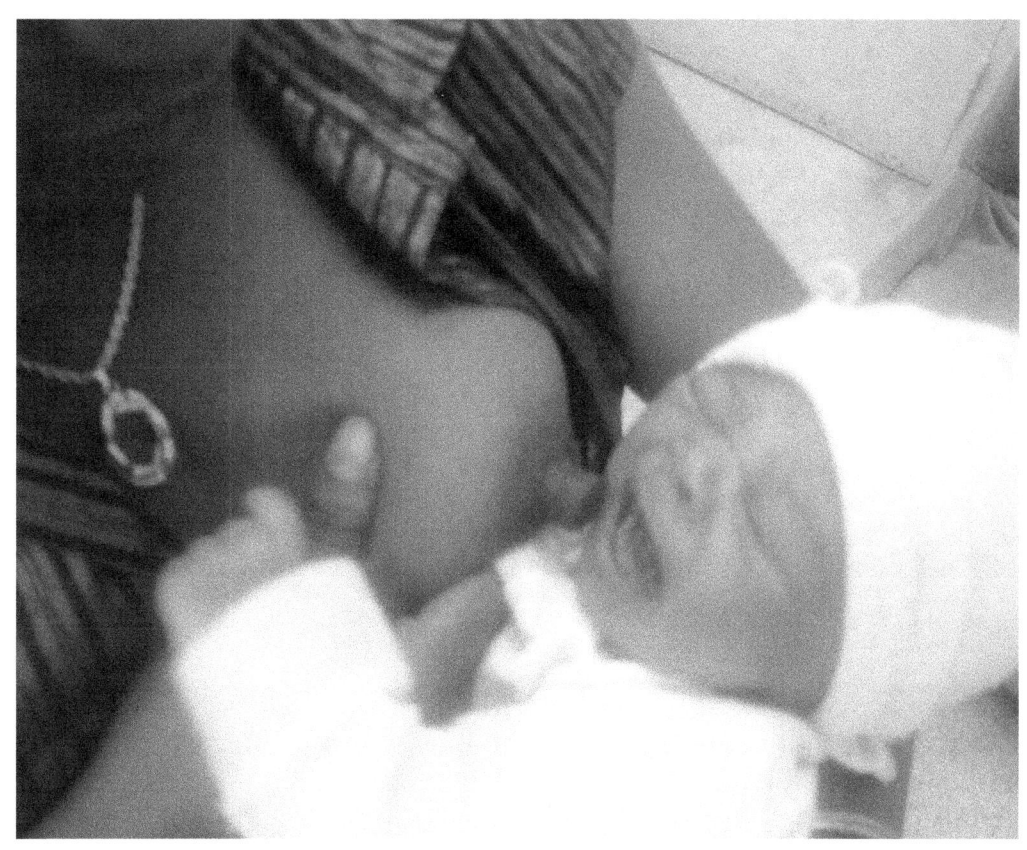

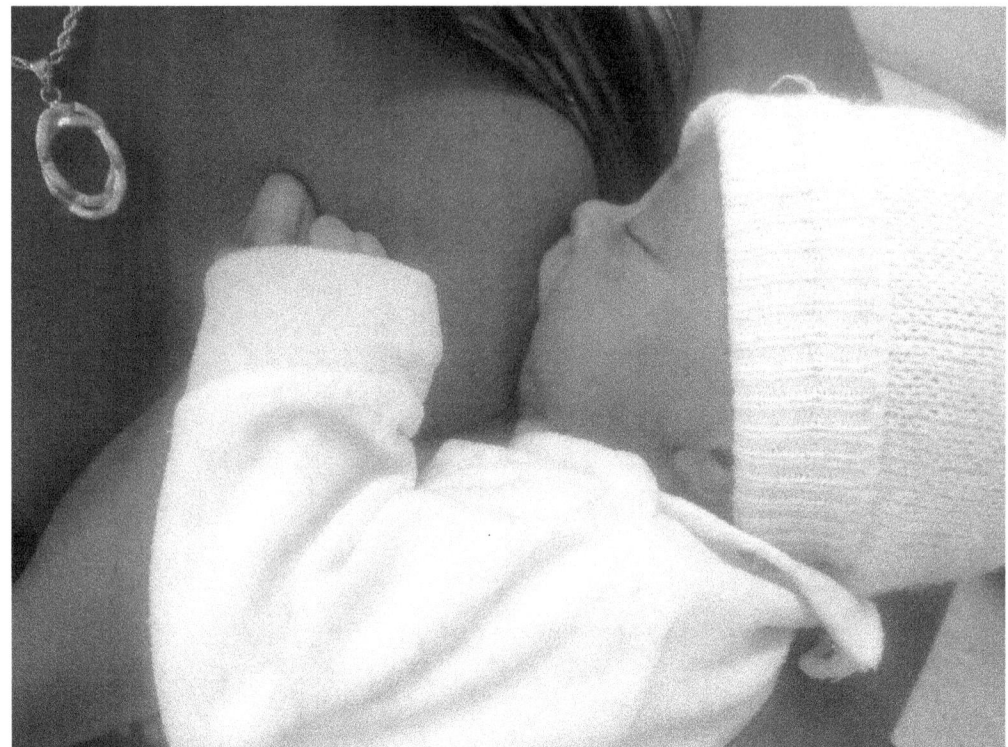

10

TONGUE TIE

One of the requests that mothers make when they visit a doctor is that the base of the tongue be cut because it is tied to the floor of the mouth and therefore the baby will not be able to talk when it grows up. Usually in the village setting the frenulum is cut with a sharp razor 'to free the tongue from the base of the mouth so that the baby can talk.

Although tongue tie can occur, it is a very rare occurrence and makes it practically difficult for the baby to suck on the breast because the tongue is needed not only to hold the breast firmly but also to swallow effectively.

Most of the babies that mothers request this operation to be carried out on are really normal babies feeding well from birth and therefore do not have tongue tie

It should be noted that most children are dumb because they cannot hear. Speech is acquired when a baby naturally tries to mimic what he hears adults around him speak.

The second reason is that the part of the brain that controls speech has been damaged much earlier by conditions like meningitis and jaundice.

Cutting the frenulum is not necessary, causes the baby unnecessary discomfort and is a potential route of introducing infection including tetanus.

Mothers should seek medical advice if they feel strongly that the tongue has a problem.

11

JAUNDICE

Jaundice is the yellow discoloration of the skin and the sclera (the white of the eye) that occurs in some disease conditions. It can occur in all age groups especially in diseases involving the liver. However here we are considering jaundice in the new born.

Jaundice occurs in a high proportion of babies within the first week of life. It is usually as a result of the accumulation of the breakdown products of blood in the circulation of the baby.

Under normal conditions the human blood cells are broken down and reproduced every three months. In other words the lifespan of a red blood cell is about 120 days. The product of this breakdown of the blood cell is called bilirubin and has a yellow colour. The liver excretes this product into the intestine and it is passed out in the stool, hence normally the healthy person does not have jaundice.

In the new born baby the liver is not mature enough to handle bilirubin in the first few days of life and it accumulates in the body of the baby making it to have a yellow skin colour. But that is not the major problem; bilirubin when the levels are high enough can enter into the brain causing irreversible damage. Some of the affected babies die while others are left with some handicaps that medical science has no way of reversing or curing.

Other causes of jaundice include infections, some blood abnormalities especially in the males, ingestion of some types of drugs, use of camphor balls to store babies and mothers' clothes and a combination of some types of blood groups.

Some of the mentally subnormal people that beg along our streets, cripples, and handicapped children in our special schools were babies that had jaundice early in life. This means that jaundice should be treated with all seriousness till it is cleared.

Jaundiced babies can be treated with exposure to the proper type of light that can clear the jaundice if it is still mild. This is called phototherapy and is carried out in many of our hospitals in Nigeria.

I have seen many babies being treated by exposure to early morning sunlight as a form of treatment. This is NOT advisable and actually endangers the life of the child. A child receiving light treatment (phototherapy) needs to be under the light

24 hours a day except when feeding. This of course cannot be achieved by the use of sunlight.

Babies with more severe jaundice can be treated by exchanging their blood with a donors' blood in a procedure called Exchange Blood Transfusion. This reduces the level of bilirubin in the baby's blood and also drastically reducing the likelihood of brain damage.

Most babies do well if they present early for treatment. Mothers are advised to see their doctor preferably a paediatrician as soon as they notice the baby has jaundice. This will also help to carry out investigations early enough for the other causes of jaundice and treat accordingly.

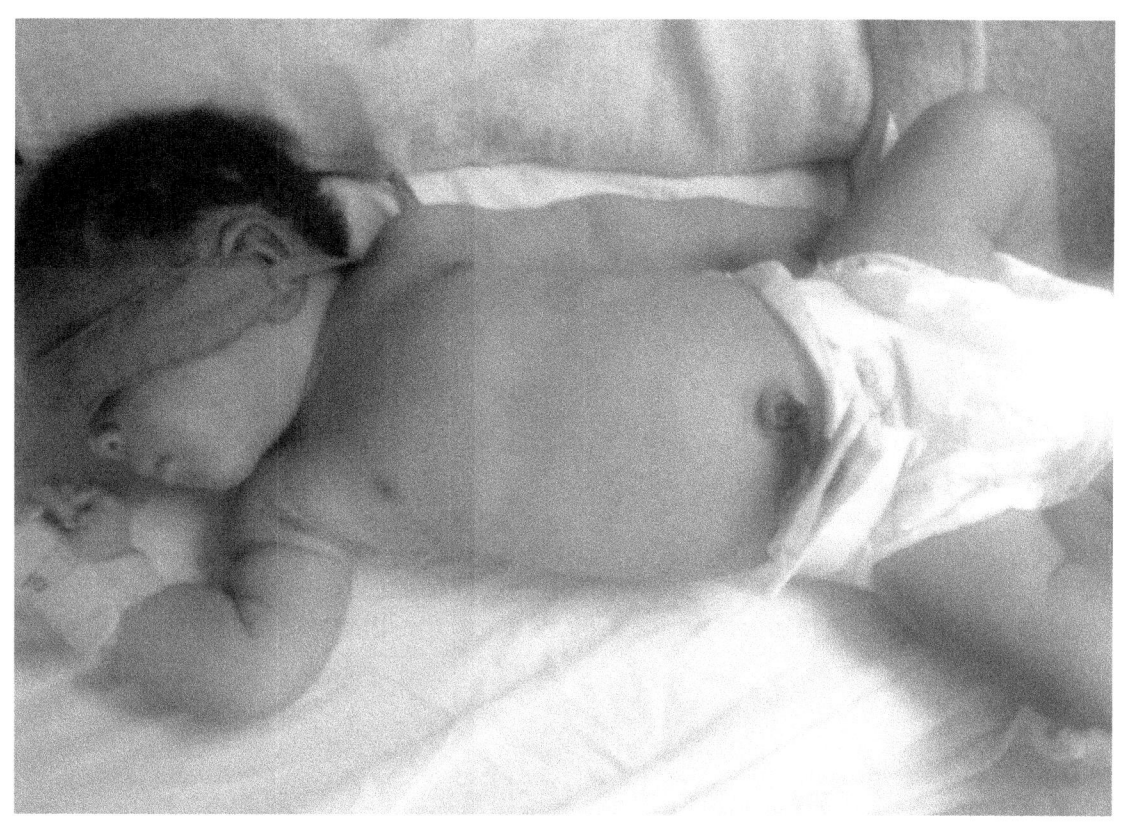

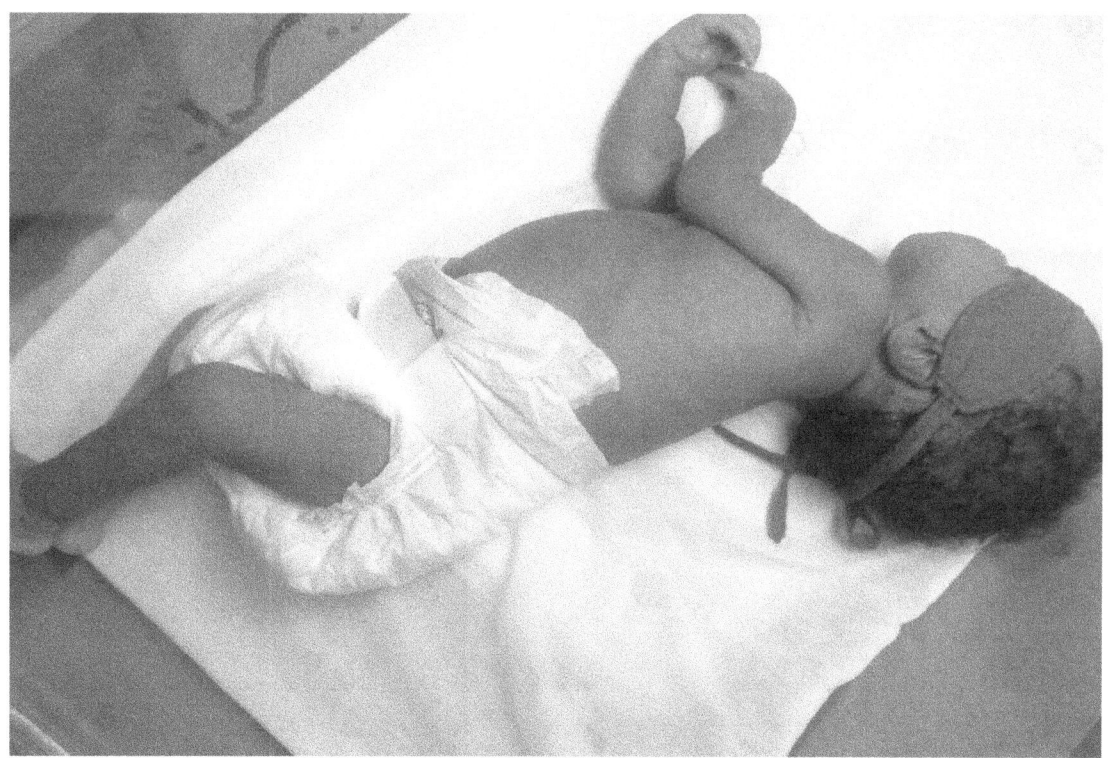

12

LOCALIZED SWELLINGS ON THE HEAD

Sometimes mothers are worried about localized swelling of the head of the baby seen soon after birth. It is mainly seen at the back and sides of the head.

These swellings are of two types, one is caused by pressure on the part of the head that comes out first and is due to pressure on that part of the head. The other is seen when delivery is assisted by the use of some instruments like the forceps or vacuum delivery. This second is usually due to accumulation of blood under the tissues of the scalp.

In both cases *nothing should be done; the swelling should be left alone* as they both regress with time and disappear.

Some people try to treat this by using hot water or in some cases drain the blood underneath. This is not necessary and could actually introduce infection into the swelling. This can result in very serious illness for the baby causing more harm than good.

13

WEAKNESS OF AN UPPER LIMB
(ERB'S PALSY AND KLUMPKE'S PARALYSIS)

Some babies go through very difficult delivery usually because they are big in size (Usually babies weighing 4kg and above). While delivering one or both shoulders a lot of pull is applied over the babies shoulder and this damages the nerves controlling the muscles of the upper limb. The affected limb is limp and not as active as the other limb if both limbs are not affected.

The best preventive measure for this condition is actually to deliver the baby detected while in the womb to be big by caesarean section.
However if this has already occurred the affected limb should not be tampered with. It is rested for at least a period of about 2-3weeks and then treated with physiotherapy. Trying to massage the limb or apply hot water worsens the damage already done and could cost the baby use of the affected limb in future.

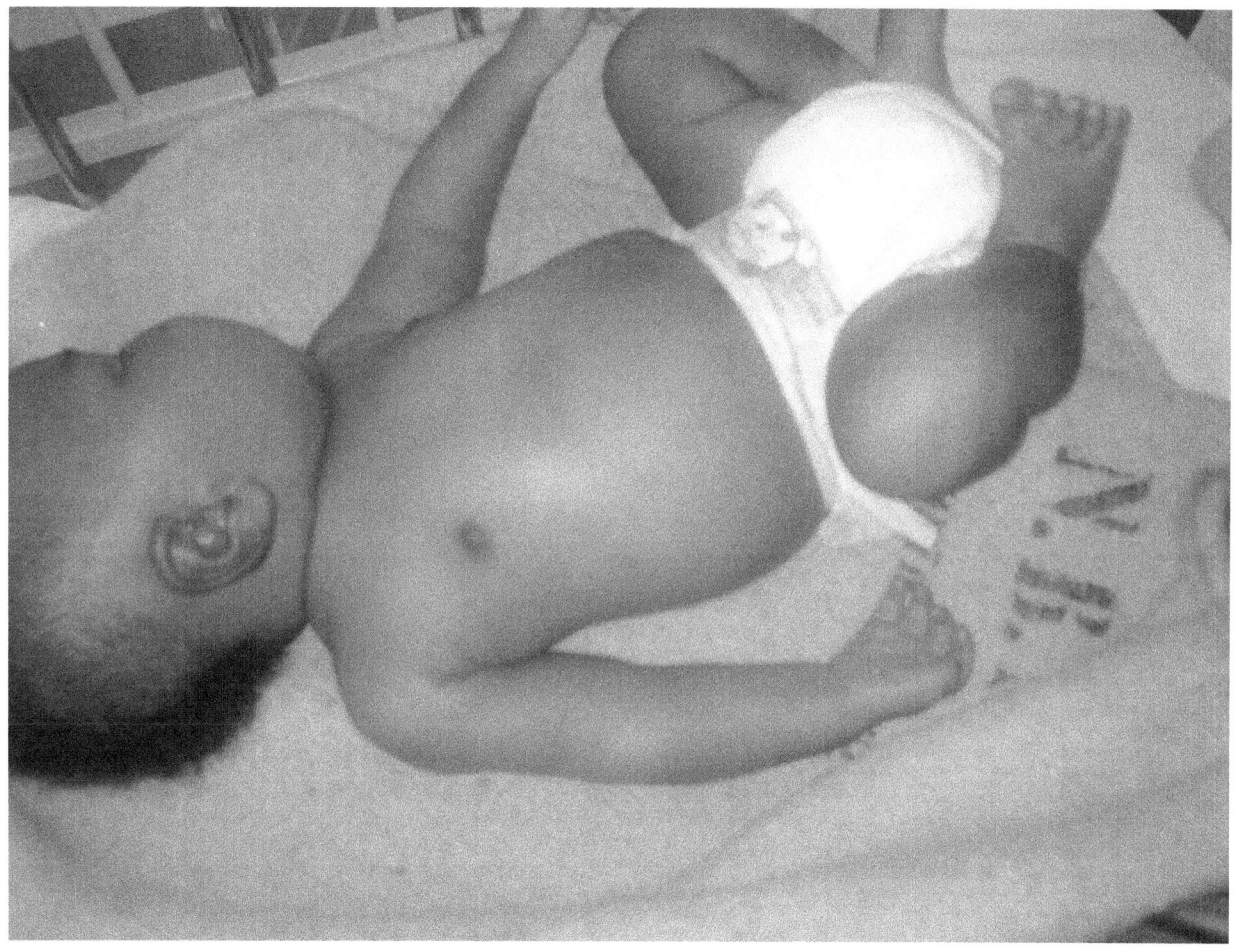

14

FRACTURE OF THE CLAVICLE

Sometimes during a difficult delivery pressure on the shoulder can cause a fracture of the clavicle (collar bone). Initially this damage is not apparent but after a few days or couple of weeks, a hard swelling appears at the middle of the collar bone which may at that time no longer be painful.

Mothers are worried about this swelling and this may be the only reason they bring the child to hospital. However nothing needs to be done about this swelling which disappears after some time. The swelling which is called callus (new bone) is actually a sign that the bone is already healing and should not be tampered with. Again it should not be massaged or treated with hot water or balms. It should be left alone.

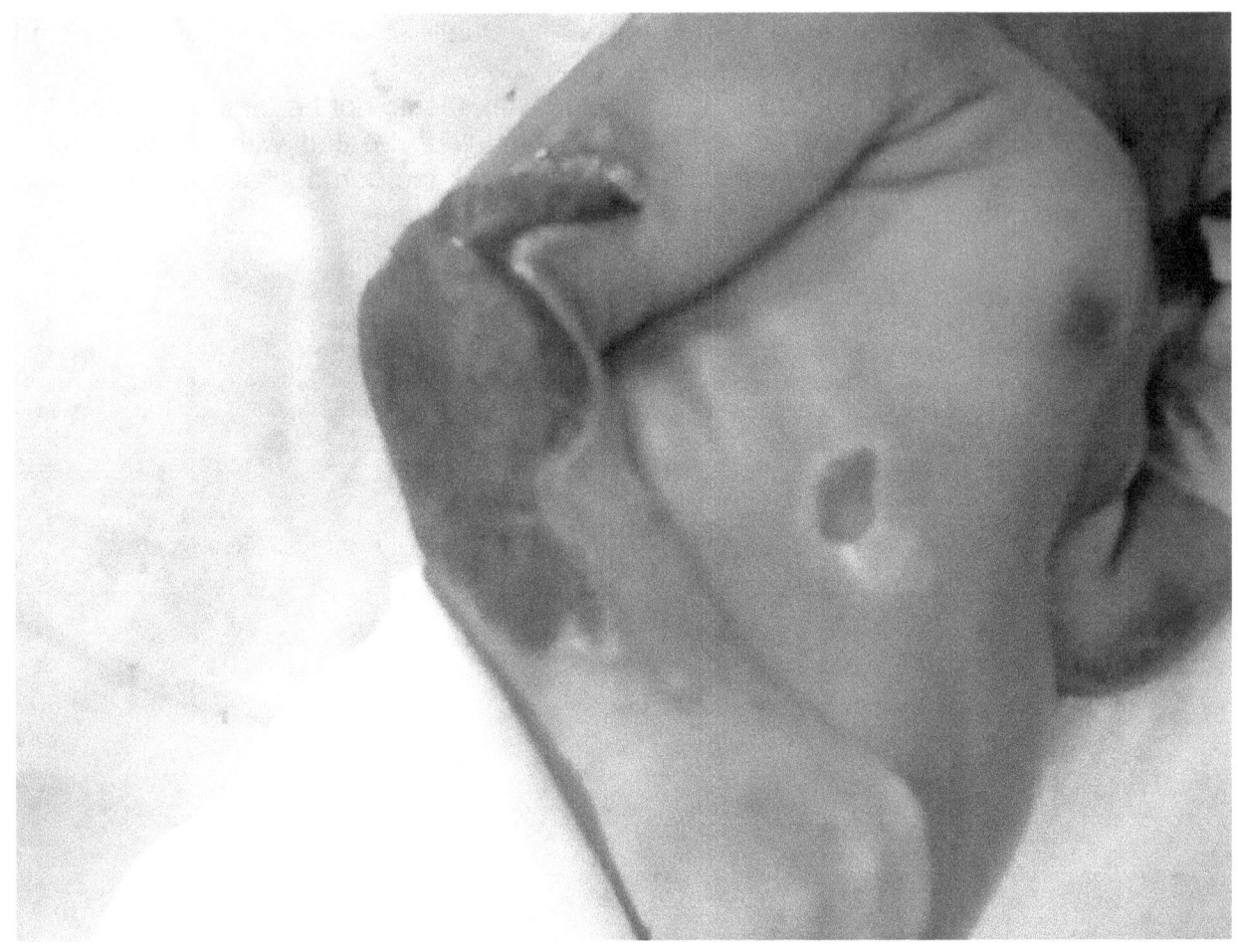

15

BREECH DELIVERY AND
BLUE COLOUR OF THE LOWER LIMBS

Not all babies delivered come out with the head first as is the case with normal deliveries; in some cases they come out with the buttocks first. This is more common with twin deliveries because of the position they assumed while in the womb. One comes out with the head first while the other comes out with the buttocks first or breech presentation.

There is absolutely nothing wrong with a baby delivered breech as the babies develop normally after delivery. It is neither a taboo nor a bad omen.

Because of the pressure applied on the buttocks during the birth process the colour of the lower limbs may remain bluish for a few days after birth. This bluish colour fades after a few days as the limbs regain their normal colour and should not be a cause of anxiety to anyone.

16

RASHES AND PEELING OF THE SKIN

In some babies that stayed a little longer than they should in the womb (post mature babies) it may be noticed that the skin appears rough and in many areas is peeling off while the nails are overgrown and the hair a little coarse. These should not be a cause of concern as these features normalize after a few days.

Many new born babies develop different types of rashes quite early in life. The most common is heat rash which appears mainly on the neck and trunk of the baby. Mothers are sometimes over protective and cover their babies from 'cold' even under the hot sun. This makes them develop rashes which is prone to secondary infection by bacteria. Babies should be exposed or be dressed with very light clothing in hot weather. If a mother is feeling hot then most likely the baby does not need to be covered.

Rashes are also common in the perineal part of the body usually due to reaction to diapers, or leaving a baby to stay too long with a wet diaper before changing it. Urine having contact with the body for too long may cause a reaction in form of rashes. Petroleum jelly can applied to protect the skin at esc change of the diapers to avoid this type of rash.

In some cases rashes develop white tips or cream coloured eruptions containing some watery fluid. This is an indication that the rash is already infected and should be treated immediately before it spreads further. The mother should consult a doctor for proper treatment. Such rash when neglected or not properly treated can lead to life threatening generalized infections.

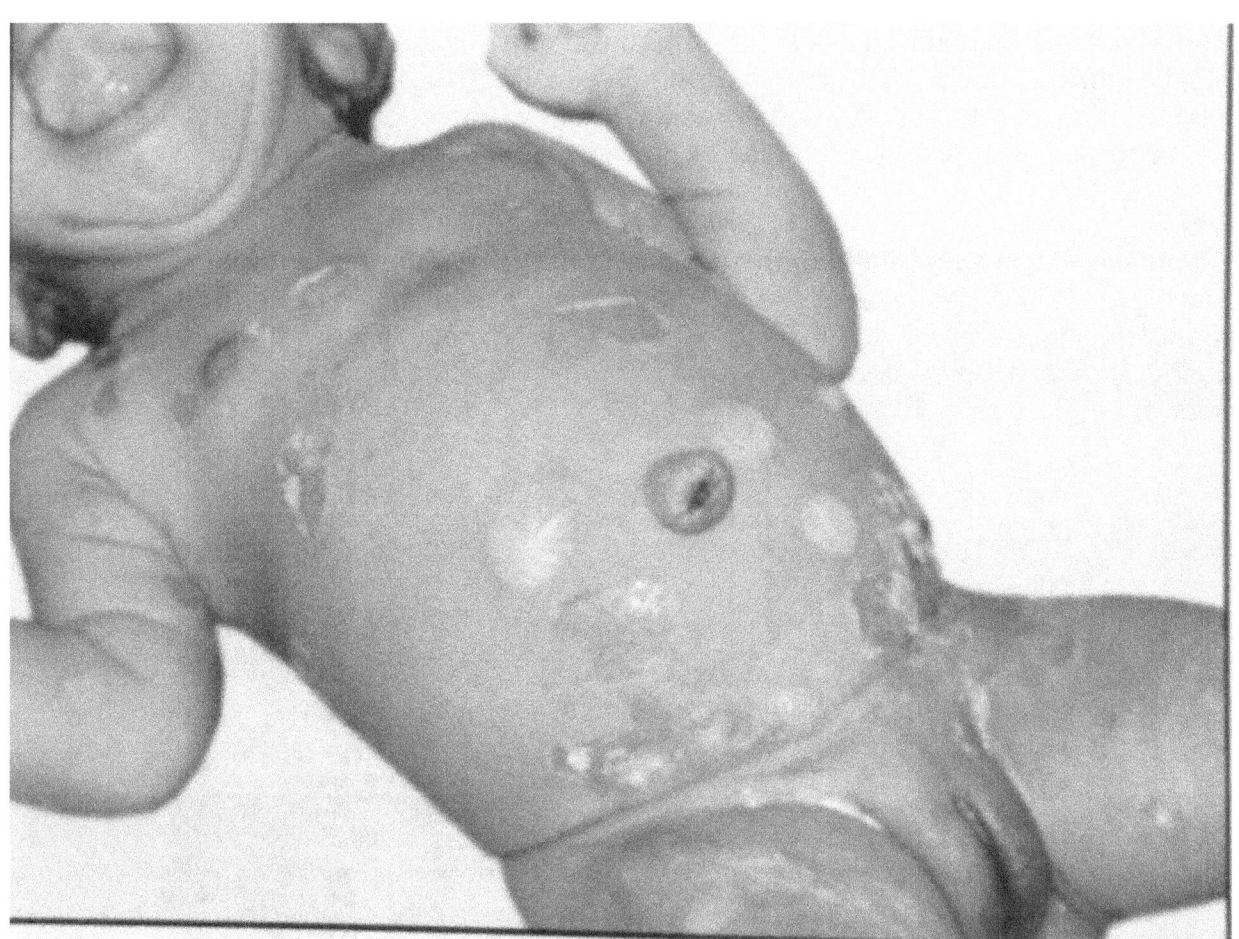

17

THE UMBILICAL STUMP

The umbilicus is the remnant of the umbilical stump which connected the baby to the mother while in the womb. It is the source of nutrition to the baby through the mother while in the womb. Apart from nutrition, oxygen, proteins conferring immunity and a lot of other factors are transferred to the baby while in the womb.

At birth the umbilicus is cut and clamped and it is necessary that the umbilical stump is treated properly so that it does not become a route of infection to the baby. Several life threatening infections including the dreadful tetanus can be contracted this way.
In hospitals, the stump is secured with a sterile clamp which is left in place until the umbilicus falls off. Where clamps are not available, a new blade can be used to cut the umbilicus while the end is securely tied with a new thread or better still a sterile suture.

The umbilical stump should be cleaned several times a day (at least 5 times) with methylated spirit and sterile gauze or cotton wool. After cleaning it should be left to dry and left open without any dressing. Creams and jellies should not be applied even if they are said to be antibacterial or antibiotic.

Some mothers are worried when the umbilical stump stays for too long before falling off. Most umbilical stumps fall off within one week of birth but some may stay for much longer but ultimately fall off. I usually ask mothers worried about this whether they have ever seen an adult still carrying his/her umbilical stump and this question usually allays their anxiety.

Sometimes even when the stump has fallen off, the surface does not heal completely leaving a whitish fleshy area the fails to dry up completely. This is called *umbilical granuloma* and may be there for several weeks causing anxiety to the mother. This fleshy area can be treated by chemically burning it off with silver nitrate sticks by a doctor.

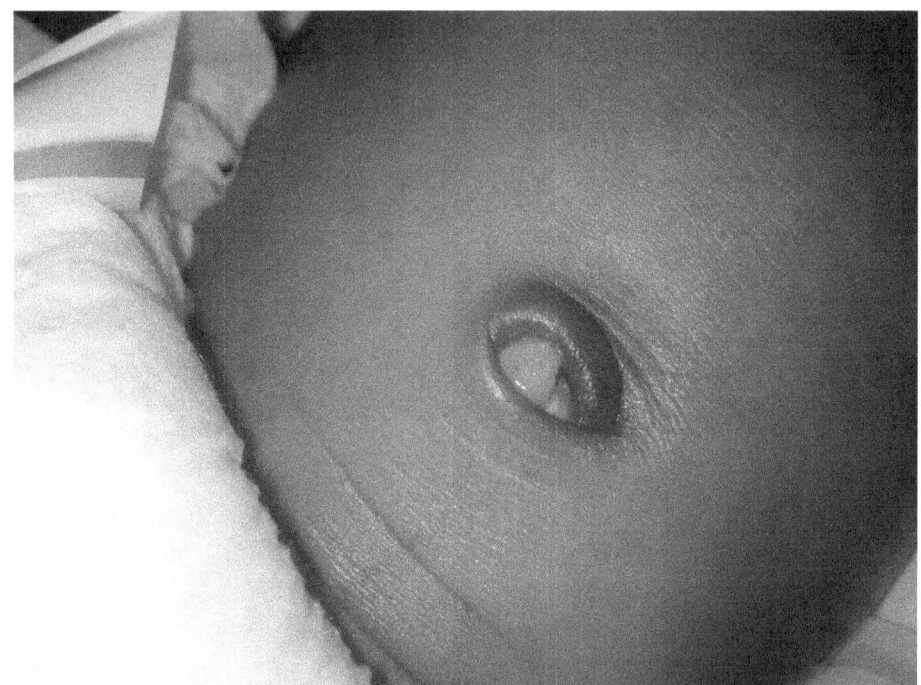

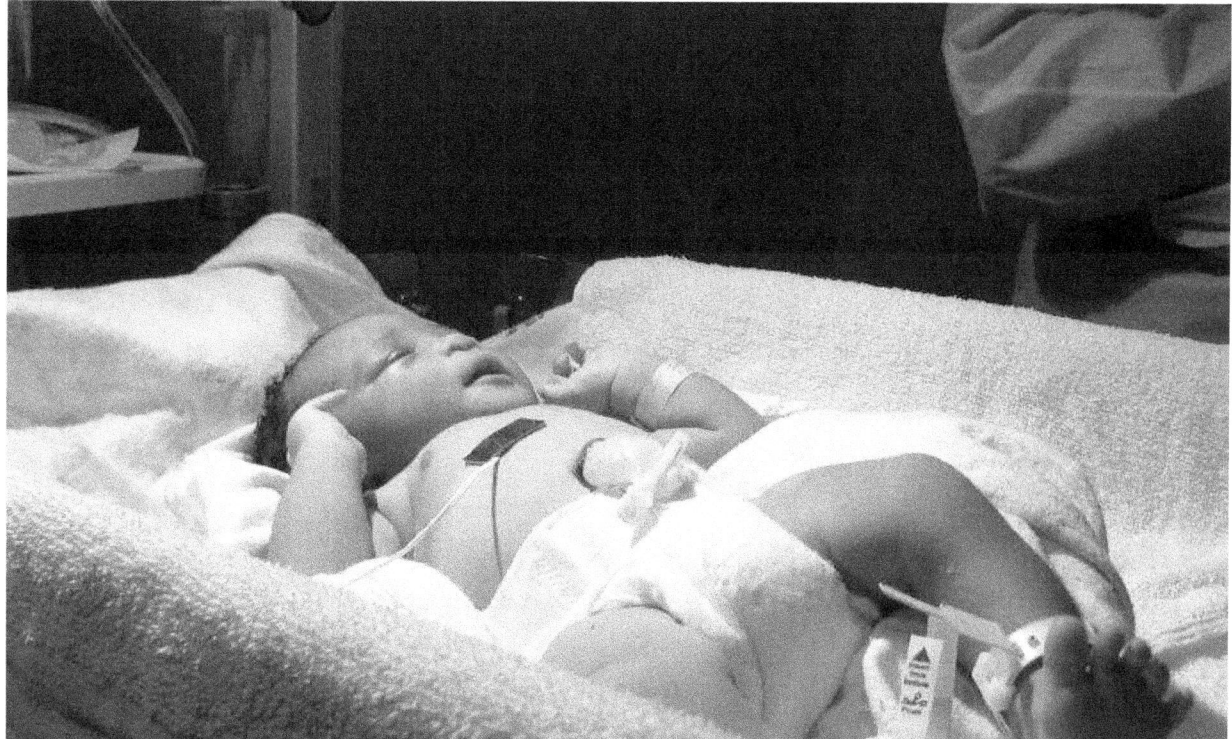

NEWBORN BABY WITH FRESH UMBILICAL STUMP. NOTICE THE CLAMP USED TO SECURE THE STUMP.

18

BOWEL HABIT, CONSTIPATION AND DIARRHOEA

The first stool a new born baby passes is usually dark green in colour and is called meconium. The time of passage of this stool varies and can be from soon after birth to 4-5 days after birth. Non passage of stools after this time should be taken seriously and requires the attention of a doctor especially when associated with abdominal distension.

The normal stool of a baby is usually golden yellow in colour and semi formed. The bowel habits of babies vary. Some babies pass stools 3-4 times daily while some babies especially those exclusively breast fed may pass stools only once in four days. This is not constipation in the real sense of it. The fact is that breast milk is almost totally absorbed in the baby's gut leaving very little to be passed out as stool. Mothers should not be worried about this.

Real constipation usually happens when a baby has been started on artificial feeds and cereals. The stools are hard and sometimes are difficult to pass out and actually make the baby to cry after much straining. To avoid this, the baby should be given enough water after feeds. If this does not help the baby can be given diluted fresh fruit juice like expressed fresh orange juice to soften the stools.

Diarrhoea or blood stained stools should be taken seriously and require medical advice and intervention. Diarrhoea occurs when a baby's stool becomes watery and more motions are passed than is usually the case. Mothers can start the baby with diarrhoea on Oral Rehydration Solution if they know how to prepare it even before seeing the doctor. ORS sachets should be handy at all times in the home so that treatment of diarrhoea can be started when need be before seeing the doctor.

19

ENLARGEMENT OF THE BREASTS
(NEONATAL MASTITIS)

The breasts of some babies start to enlarge some weeks or even days after birth and some mothers on the advice of relations or friends decide to express them.Some look like the breasts of young girls approaching puberty. They, according to the informants contain milk (so called witches milk) or pus and are supposed to be expressed and thrown away. In some cases hot water compresses are applied occasionally leading to burns. In some cases some people think that this is actually an abscess and try to incise them.

This information is not accurate. What actually happens is that the hormones that the mother produced during pregnancy crosses into the baby's circulation and after birth stimulates the tissues of the baby's breasts to enlarge just like the mother's. The breasts are not actually infected and need no treatment. Expressing or incising them can actually now lead to infection of the tissues which has to be vigorously treated.

The breasts should be left alone and not tampered with. After some time, when these hormonal levels get reduced the breasts return to their normal size

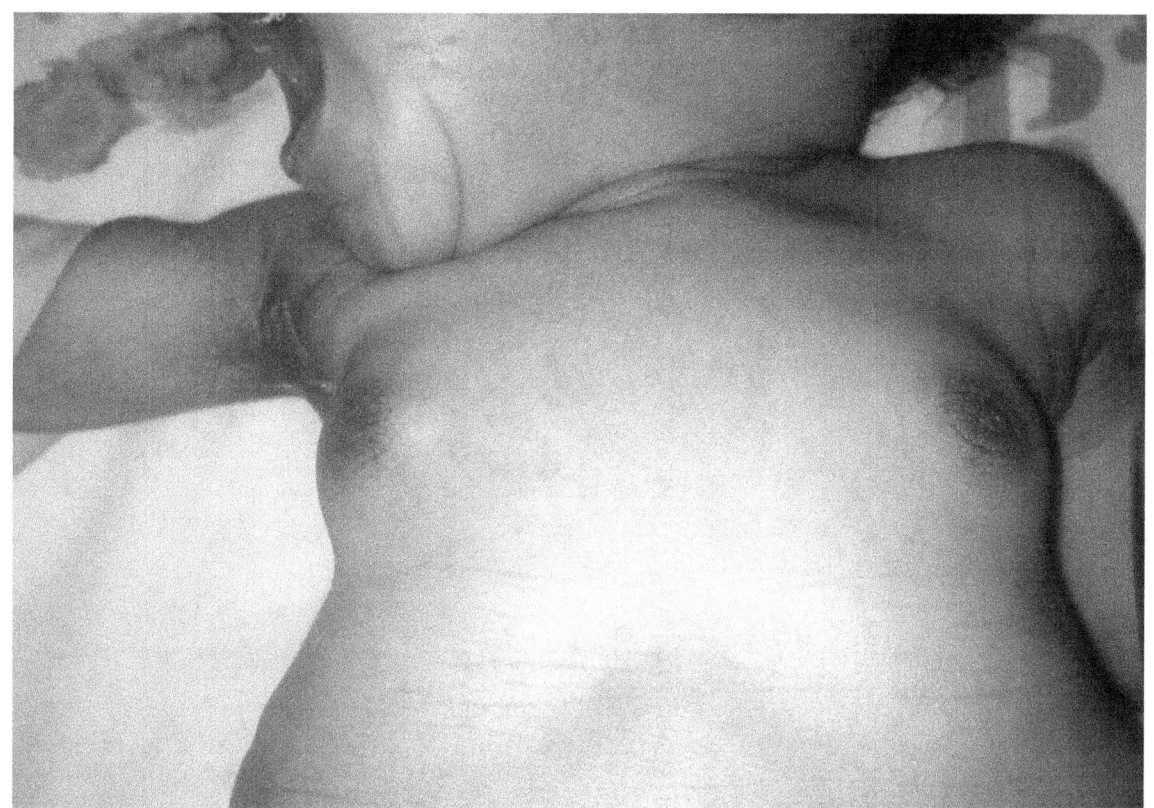

20

SLEEPING PROBLEMS

The sleeping pattern of babies is different from that of a normal adult. Many babies sleep a lot during the day but wake up several times in the night to breast feed. The different demands of each baby are different and will be understood by the mother as time goes on.

Most babies sleep most of the time only waking up to feed or when the diapers are wet. Some mothers complain about the baby not sleeping enough in the night because of the number of times they need to wake and feed the child forgetting that the baby had been sleeping almost all day. This is not really a problem as the baby gradually adjusts to the sleeping pattern of adults as he develops.

One of the things that make babies cry a lot is improper feeding by the mothers. Some babies are prone to sleeping when they are put on the breast and they therefore sleep off before they are full. Because of this, after sleeping for a short time they wake up again from hunger and start to cry. The mother feeds once more and the baby is not satisfied before sleeping off and wakes up soon after. The cycle continues and the mother who then does not have much rest gets frustrated. If the baby sleeps off while feeding he may need to be woken up to finish his feeding. A well fed baby usually sleeps for three or more hours before waking up again thereby giving the mother enough time not only to rest but also do some other things.

However, if a baby does not sleep much during the day and also in the night, despite good feeding, medical attention should be sought especially when this is associated with poor weight gain or even weight loss. Causes may include some infections including malaria in our environment and should be properly treated.

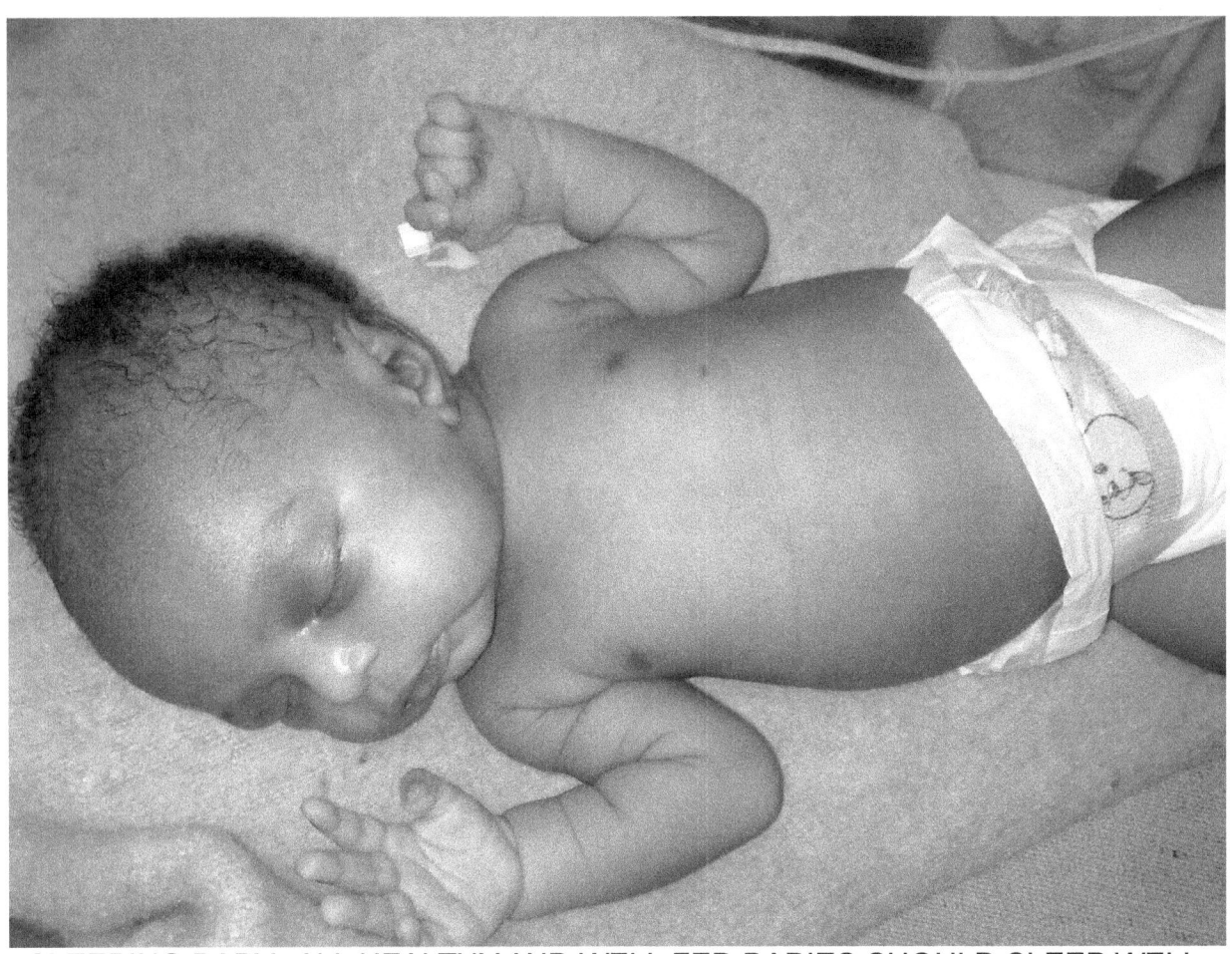

SLEEPING BABY. ALL HEALTHY AND WELL FED BABIES SHOULD SLEEP WELL.

TEETHING AND FEVERS

There is a general misconception in different cultures about the association of teething with some symptoms of ill health especially fevers and diarrhoea. Most people believe that teething is associated with fevers and loose stools and sometimes vomiting and general malaise. The danger of this belief is that babies are left at home without seeking for medical attention until the condition gets very bad or it is even too late.

Every baby acquires immunity to many disease conditions while in the mothers' womb as has been mentioned before. These are in form of proteins called immune globulins that are passed on to the child through the placenta. These proteins help to fight different diseases like malaria, chicken pox, measles and different types of diarrhoeal diseases.

However the baby's body systems are not yet mature enough to generate these proteins on their own and as the baby grows within the first few months the levels begin to drop making the child prone to different types of infections.

At the age of 4-5 months the baby now starts to have infections like malaria, viral diarrhoea, different types of pneumonias and some other viral infections that are difficult to identify clinically. He now comes down with more frequent attacks of fever. It is also at this time that the teeth start to erupt and the fevers are wrongly attributed to teething. When these babies are properly attended to medically the fever subsides but the teeth continue to erupt; if eruption causes the fever it should have continued even with treatment.

Teething powders are mainly made from analgesic tablets crushed to a powder form. They may give relief for the fever temporarily but the underlying disease condition is not eliminated and may actually be incubating in the baby's body making the condition potentially worse.

Any baby that has a fever should be properly treated since there are numerous causes of fever many of which can be potentially fatal. Proper investigations should be carried out where necessary and appropriate treatment given. In most cases, when this is done the cause of the fever is detected.

EAR DISCHARGE/INFECTIONS

Ear infections are common in the first year of life and can be a source of anxiety and frustration for a mother. The ear is usually infected through the throat because the ear is connected to the throat by the canal called the Eustachian tube. This tube is usually angulated in the adult but straight in the baby. Any infection in the throat of the baby can therefore easily be transmitted into the middle ear. Most ear infections are therefore preceded by a throat infection which may not be noticeable by the mother.

The baby with ear infection cries inconsolably and all the mother's methods of pacifying the child, breast feeding, giving water, rocking the baby all fail to stop the baby from crying. This is despite the fact that no obvious cause of the problem may be seen – no swellings, many a time no fever, no rash etc. I have seen not a few of these mothers bring their babies to the hospital also crying with the baby, having failed in getting the baby to stop crying.

The tension created in the middle ear (which has no space for expansion) is the cause of the severe pain. Sometimes when appropriate treatment is not offered the ear membrane (tympanic membrane) ruptures oozing out pus as ear discharge; the baby is relieved and now cries less but the problem is not yet over.

The infection may become chronic and damage the hearing organs inside the ear leading to deafness of the affected ear. The middle ear is also very close to the brain and infection could cross into the brain causing meningitis or brain abscess; both very serious causes of morbidity and mortality.

Any baby that cries more than the mother is used to should be taken to see the doctor for proper evaluation.

There is a misconception that mothers lying down to breast feed their babies is the cause of ear infection. This is far from the truth and is based on the assumption that the ear discharge has a similar colour with the breast milk. Mothers can breast feed their babies lying down so far as the baby is well latched on to the breast and can feed properly.

23

ABDOMINAL GRIPES AND REGURGITATION OF FEEDS

This is a common problem that brings some babies to hospital. The mother complains that the baby is always writhing in pain especially after feeding. This sometimes disturbs sleep at night and the parents are worried.

Some people attribute this to readjustment of abdominal organs after birth and problems with the umbilicus and the navel especially when the baby has umbilical hernia. This is not necessarily so.

Oftentimes abdominal gripes are caused by a lot of gas in the babies' gut mainly due to two major reasons. When the baby is not properly positioned (latched to the breast) while feeding, he may swallow a lot of air while feeding.
Secondly if the baby is not properly bopped (rubbing the back until he belches) after feeding there is a lot of swallowed air in the abdomen that makes the baby uncomfortable and can also lead to regurgitation of the feed given. This can be likened to the feeling when we have indigestion after taking half done or stale food.

Babies should be bopped properly after each feed until they belch to avoid regurgitation and abdominal gripes.

Some remedies are usually applied for this purpose including the popular gripe water. In my own opinion, some of the contents of these remedies are not well spelt out or contain nothing that can help the child. They should therefore be avoided. Mild antacids, where the measures mentioned above do not work can be used to make the child more comfortable.

After feeding, when the baby sleeps off he should be placed lying in a prone position with the face turned to one side to avoid regurgitation and possible aspiration of the feed which can be dangerous.

Persistent abdominal pain, especially when associated with vomiting and abdominal distension requires urgent medical intervention.

24

VAGINAL DISCHARGE

This of course applies to only female babies. Some days after delivery the mother notices some thick creamy white discharge from the vagina and this of course frightens her because she attributes it to an infection (Sexually transmitted diseases type). Some actually come to the hospital complaining that they do not know how their baby contracted such infection.

Some babies actually go as far as having a bloody discharge which of course is very frightening to the parents.

This should not actually be a source of anxiety. As explained for neonatal mastitis these discharges are caused by the effect of maternal hormones which had crossed into the baby's circulation causing the discharge and bleeding (like menstrual flow). There is no need for any intervention since the discharge soon stops in a couple of days.

25

CONVULSIONS AND JITTERINESS

Jitteriness occurs normally in many new born babies causing anxiety for the parents. The baby occasionally seems to tremble especially the upper limbs. This lasts for a very short time and then stops. When this is prolonged it may be a sign of low blood sugar and the baby must fed immediately. Low blood sugar can lead to convulsions in babies. Some babies that are given only water for the first 48 hours after delivery. This practice is not good; babies should be put to breast as soon as possible after delivery.

Babies can also startle at loud noises. Mothers get worried at this and think it is a sign of illness or seizure. This is actually a good sign as far as the doctor is concerned because it is a confirmation that the baby has good hearing.

Convulsion is however is a very serious symptom and should be treated with a sense of urgency. It could be obvious or not easily noticeable. It can also be localized or generalized and the eyes could roll up, which symptoms are very frightening to the mother. The baby should immediately be taken to the doctor for proper evaluation and treatment.

The causes of seizures in the new born are many and mothers should not presume to know what the problem is or prolong the time of intervention. Convulsions can lead to severe brain damage and should be treated with all seriousness.

35

ORAL THRUSH

Many a time some white patches are seen in themouths of new born babies liming the walls of the mouth and the tongue.They are easily cleaned off with a soft cloth or tissue paper. These patches are remnants of the breast milk that had been given to the baby.

However in some cases these patches are different, sticking to the walls of the mouth and tongue and bleeding if some force is applied to remove them. This is called oral thrush caused by fungal infection. It occurs in many babies because of their low immunity and usually disappears as the child grows without any treatment.

However, if this growth becomes excessive or persistent treatment is necessary. Oral anti-fungal drugs usually in the form of suspensions are effective and can be obtained after consulting a doctor. The use of gentian violet is very messy and no longer advised.

Any baby with longstanding oral thrush should be properly investigated as the condition can also be caused by clinical states that lower immunity.

36

BIRTH MARKS

Birth marks are areas of the skin that are not the same colour with the rest of the body. Most are dark in colour sometimes with tufts of hair, but in many babies these areas are transient and soon become the same colour with the rest of the body.

In some cases some of these areas have the colour of coffee mixed with milk and may be multiple appearing in many parts of the body as small patches. When a baby with this discoloration of the skin also has repeated episodes of convulsions, medical attention is required.

Some birthmarks are different, usually elevated to some extent and dark cherry red or bright red in colour; an indication that they contain a lot of tiny blood vessels. Many of these decrease in size until they finally disappear; some others actually increase in size and may start to bleed when the surface is eroded. These latter types need medical attention as they can ulcerate and bleed profusely; some may require the attention of a plastic surgeon for proper repair.

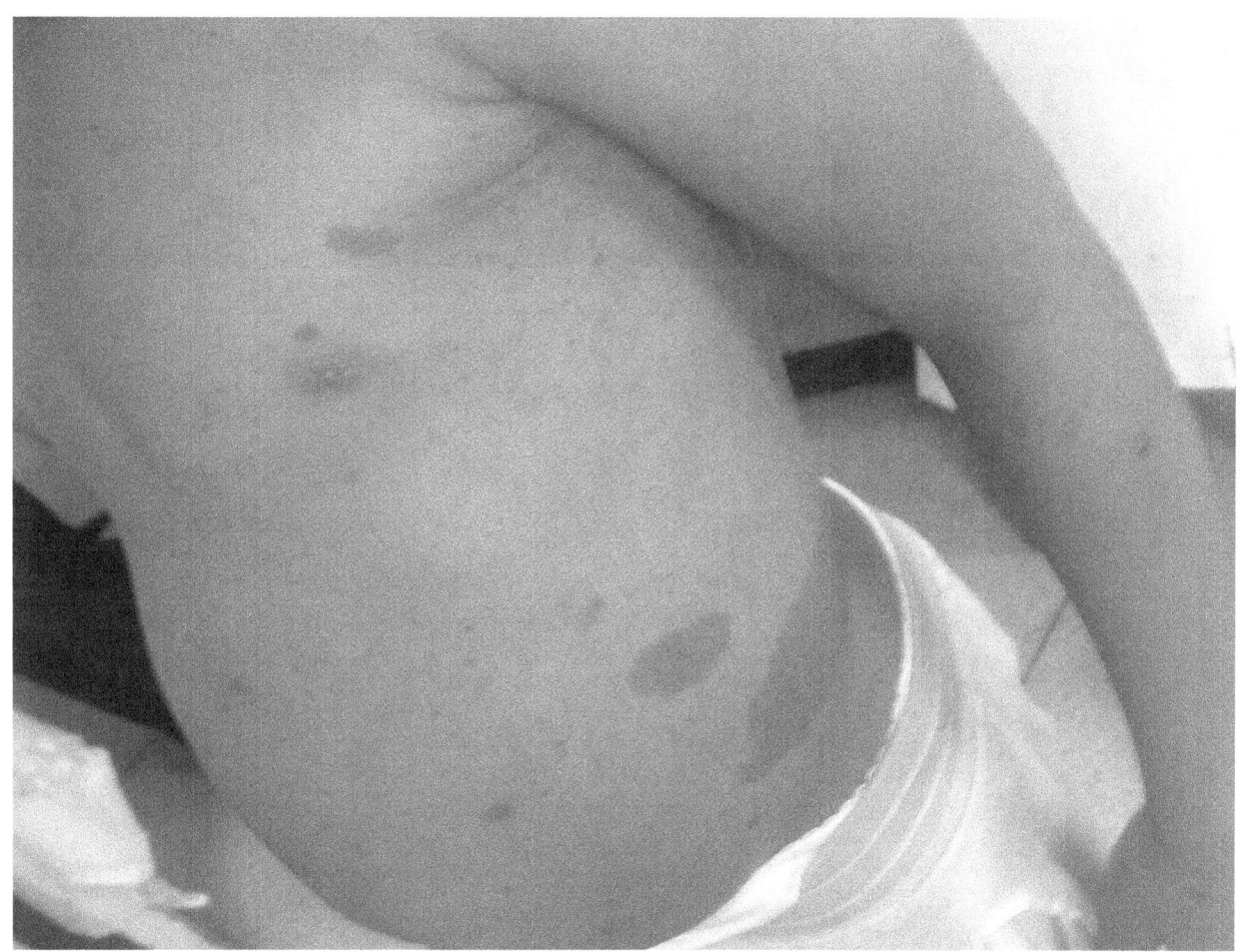

37
CIRCUMCISION

This refers only to male circumcision which should be carried out in normal male babies from the eight day of life. Circumcision before the eight day of life is not safe because the clotting mechanism of the baby is still immature at this time and the baby may bleed uncontrollably.

Two types of circumcision are available, the traditional type where the foreskin is cut off with a sharp edge and the *plastibel* type in which the foreskin is stretched over a bell-like appliance and tied firmly over it to fall off on its own later. Both procedures are good in the hands of proficient practitioners.

Circumcision should not be carried out when the sex of the baby is still in doubt; so called *ambiguous genitalia.* It should also not be carried out when the penile shaft of the baby looks abnormal, such as when the baby's urethra appears to be below instead of in front of the penis (*hypospadias*). This is because the repair of this abnormality may require the use of the foreskin and this may be difficult if the foreskin has been cut off.

Circumcision should also be delayed in babies that are premature until they get to an acceptable weight. Sick babies, babies with jaundice and babies that are deficient in some blood clotting factors should also not undergo circumcision without proper medical cover. Medical advice should be sought under these conditions.

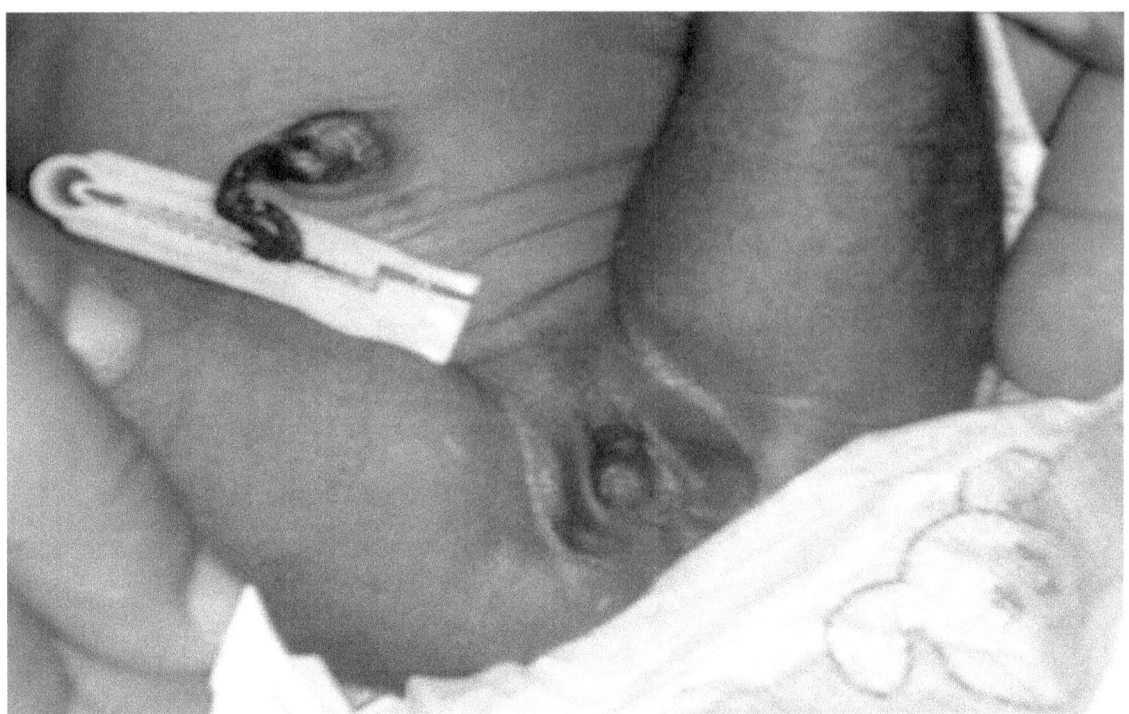

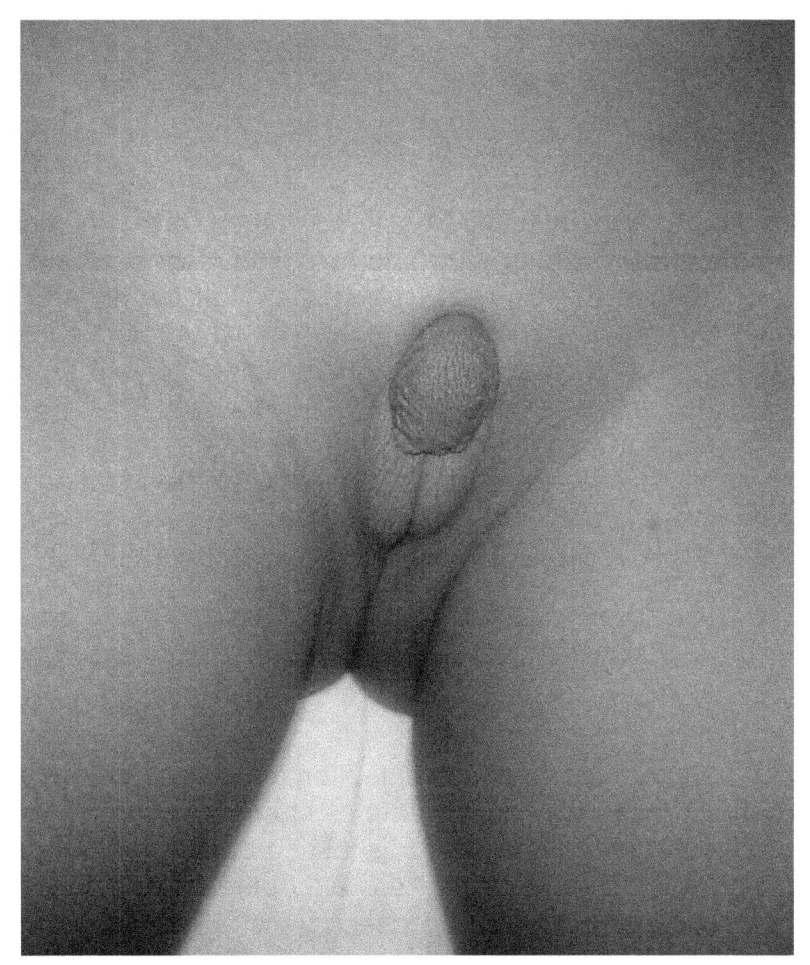

38
INFECTIONS

New born babies are prone to infections because of their low immunity and everything possible must be done to protect them from acquiring infections. Some of the infections are acquired in-utero (while the baby is still in the mothers' womb). These include syphilis, rubella (German measles), many types of viral infections including hepatitis B, retroviral infection (HIV) and other less common infections.

Other infections can be acquired during delivery when the baby is passing through the birth canal. These again include infections of the eye that lead to eye discharge after delivery (ophthalmia neonatorum). This infection can cause some damage to the eyes and can be due to infection by several organisms. HIV and hepatitis B infection can also be acquired during delivery.

After delivery, many other bacterial infections are possible including tetanus, meningitis, septicaemia (infection in the blood stream) which are all life threatening.

It is also noteworthy that most of these infections are easily preventable. Mothers should make sure they receive the immunizations in order to protect their children. The umbilical stump should be taken care of as discussed earlier. Mothers that their babies had eye discharge should make sure they are adequately treated so that subsequent babies will not have the same problem. If necessary the father should also be treated.

Some mothers start draining water (liquor) before the onset of labour sometimes for onwards of two weeks. This is a very potent source of bacterial infection to the unborn baby. The mother should be put on antibiotics prophylactically before the onset of labour to protect both the mother and the baby.

Infections can cause a lot of damage to the baby if not properly treated and some of the residual damages can be permanent especially when the brain is involved. Every effort should therefore be made to maintain good hygiene especially regular hand washing and good care of the breasts by the nursing mother. Early signs of infection like fever, refusal of feeds and weakness should therefore be taken seriously and the doctor consulted.

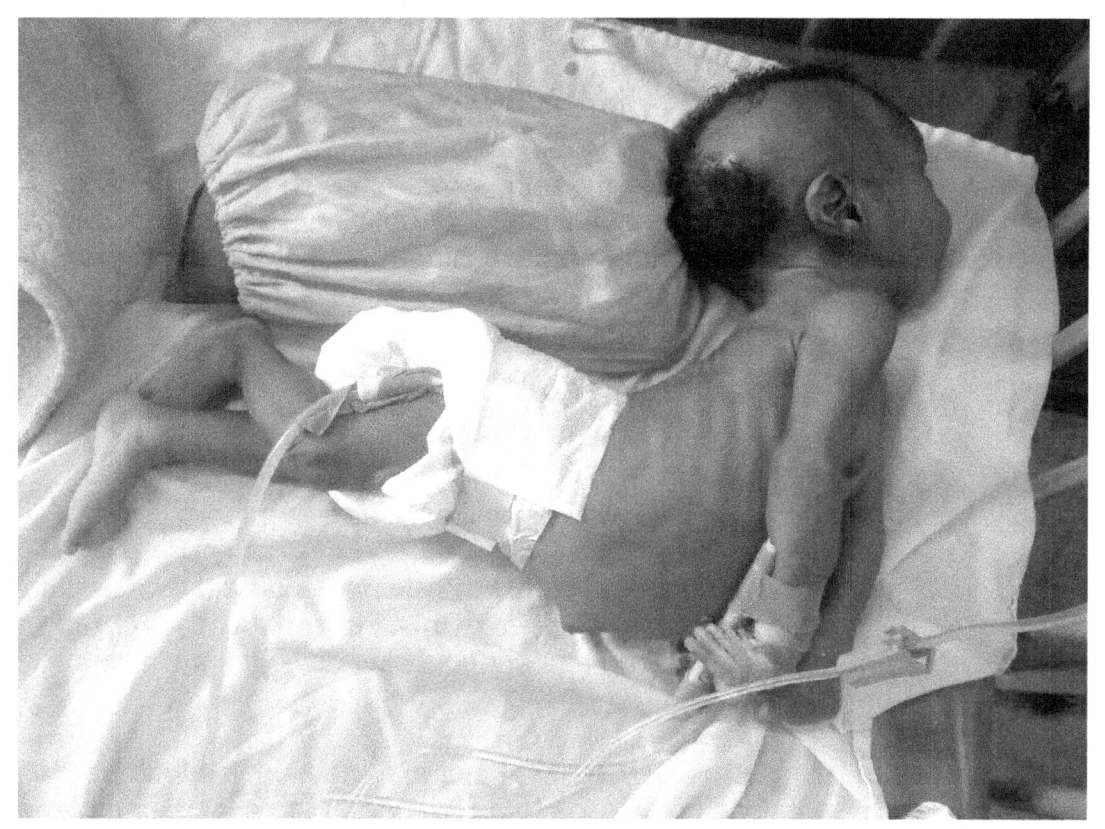

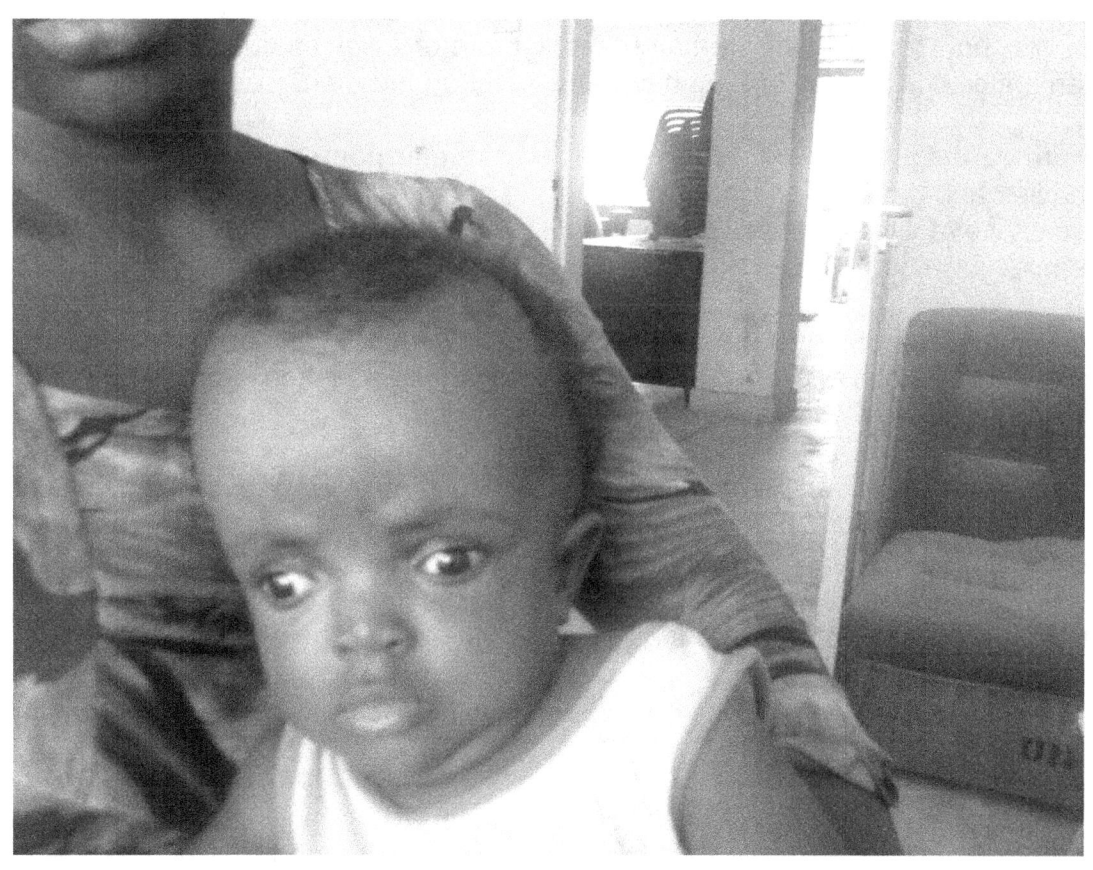

DIARRHOEA

Diarrhoea is the passage of three or more loose or watery in a 24 hour. A loose stool is the one that takes the shape of the container. This definition is adequate for the child but is difficult to justify with the neonate and the infant below the age of three months. This is because, particularly for the new born baby the stool is rather loose and may fall into the category of diarrhoea if this definition is applied.

For this group of babies diarrhoea can be said to be passage of more frequent, usually watery or loose stools more than what has hitherto been observed by the mother before.
When the stool also contains visible blood stains it is called dysentery.

Diarrhoea can be caused by various organisms, mainly bacterial and viral but the most common cause of childhood diarrhoea is the rotavirus. Bacterial causes are also very important especially the shigella, salmonella and klebsiella infections which can cause epidemics in New born units.

The real cause of death in diarrhoeal disease is not the infection itself but dehydration. The loss of fluid from the baby's body leads to a collapse of the circulatory system and subsequently death. The focus on the management of the baby with diarrhoea is therefore fluid replacement until the viral infection is burnt out, and not treatment of the cause of the infection.

Most of the diarrhoeal diseases are caused by viruses as mentioned before and viruses do not respond to antibiotic treatment. It is therefore not useful to give the affected children antibiotics as they will not have any effect on the diarrhoea.

Anti-diarrhoeal agents usually given to adults with diarrhoea and generally available in pharmacies and patent medicine shops are not useful in childhood diarrhoea. Adults do not usually have viral diarrhoea but bacterial. These anti diarrhoeals are actually meant for them.

Moreover, these anti-diarrhoeal agents slow down gut movement (motility) causing pooling of fluid in the child's gut leading to abdominal distension. Some can also cause convulsions in babies. It is not advisable to use them.

The use of oral rehydration salts in form of the solution, Oral rehydration Solution has saved the lives of millions of children in the last two decades. Two types are available,
1) The home-made preparation which contains table salt and sugar or Salt Sugar Solution (SSS)–
2) The UNICEF oral rehydration salts pre-packed in sachets (ORS)

The SSS can be prepared at home and is advised to be used only for emergencies until a proper medical consultation is obtained.

The ORS contains all the salts the child is losing in the stool and calories for energy and is therefore a balanced solution for the treatment of childhood diarrhoea. One sachet should be mixed with one Litre of water and given to the child in small aliquots that he/she can tolerate. 5-10ml at a time swallowed and retained is a lot better than a whole cup given and vomited. Vomiting also makes the child weaker, thus compounding the anxiety and fright of the mother.

TIPS

- Mothers are advised to keep a few sachets of UNICEF ORS handy at home and start using it as soon as they notice the baby has developed diarrhoea even before consulting a doctor. Acute diarrhoea that started in the night could go bad before the day breaks.

- SSS could be used in place of this as an emergency if ORS is not available before seeing the doctor

- Patience is required since it takes a few days tor the viral infection to burn out.

- Mothers should not expect the sick baby to still be taking the food as when he/she was well.

- Force-feeding the child leads to more vomiting and more frustration. Oral sips of beverages for the older child, and breast milk only for the infant is enough for the child's recovery.

- Half strength pap is also advised since the normal strength pap will only worsen the diarrhoea by a mechanism called osmotic diarrhoea.

- Solid food for the older child should be avoided at this time. It may worsen the diarrhoea

- Unfortunately most mothers believe in feeding the child his/her normal diet at this time since they believe they will recover faster.

- The new born baby can also have diarrhoea and should be treated the same way with ORS.

- ORS does not cure or stop diarrhoea as some mothers expect. It is meant to be used to replace the fluid the baby is losing until the viral infection burns out and normal bowel motion is once more established. If this is not done the child gets dehydrated.

Any child with diarrhoea with or without vomiting can deteriorate rapidly without proper intervention. Medical consultation should be sought as early as possible.

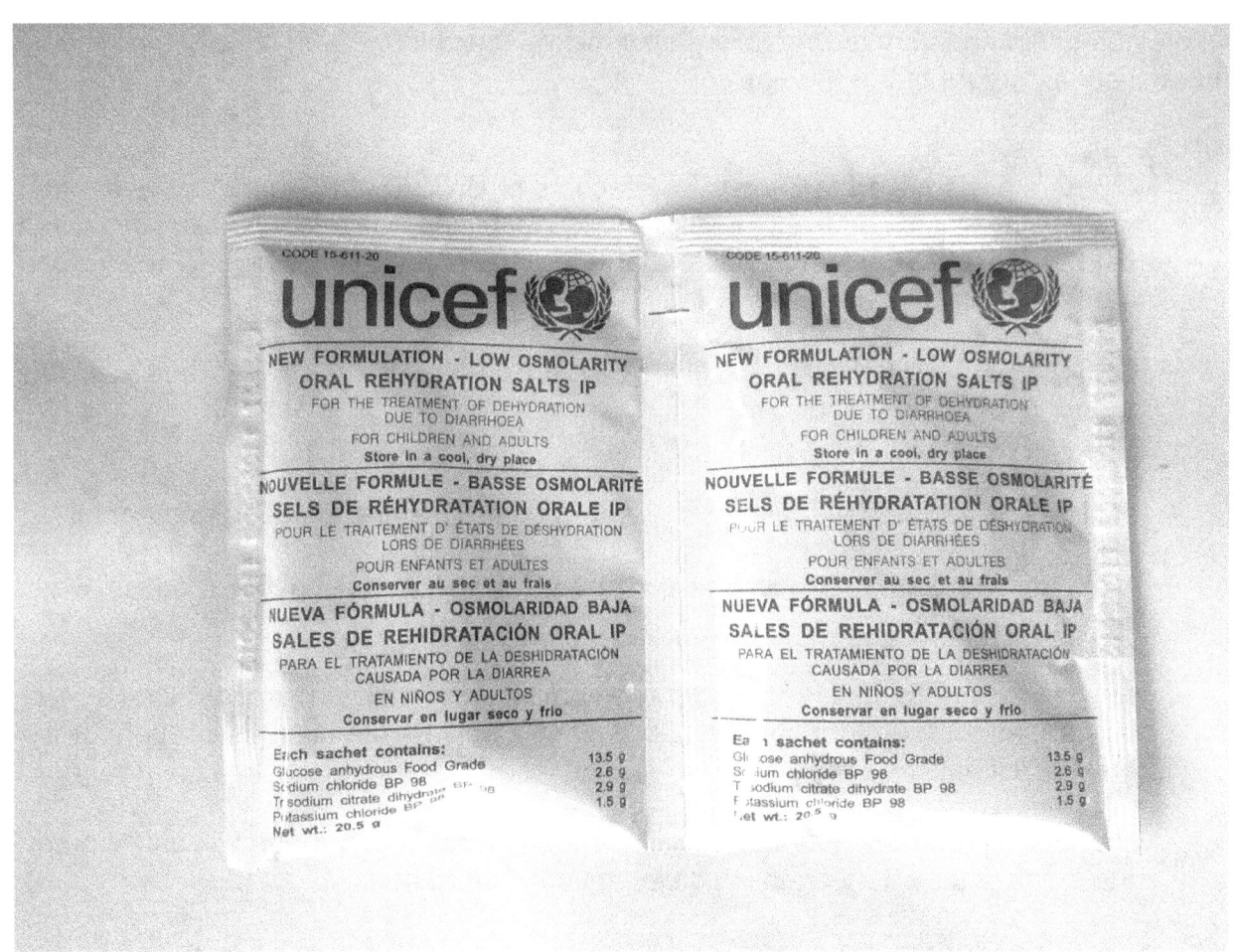

UNICEF ORT SACHETS
SHOULD ALWAYS BE HANDY AT HOME

40

PREMATURITY

A baby is said to be premature when it is delivered before the pregnancy is term, usually 40 weeks gestation. In medical circles, any baby delivered from 37-40weeks of gestation is regarded as a full term baby.

However for some reasons some babies are delivered before they are due and this is associated with several problems including the probability of survival. In our environment babies delivered from 28 weeks gestation are more likely to survive if given proper medical attention.

In developed countries, because of the advancement in medical practice, babies as low as 21 weeks gestation now survive. Any delivery before this time is not likely to survive and is regarded as an abortion.

Premature babies should ideally be nursed in a special care unit under the care of medical experts trained to handle them. They usually have problems of temperature control, feeding, infections, dehydration among others.

The most important thing to take care of in a premature baby after birth is temperature control. The baby should be wrapped in warm clothes and if possible hot water bottle can be used to keep the baby warm while being transported as quickly as possible to a specialist centre that can handle them.

A premature baby can also be kept warm by wrapping her onto the mothers' body with warm clothing so that the mothers' body heat can keep her warm. This is the so-called kangaroo nursing. If the mother is incapacitated, like mothers that delivered through caesarean section, anybody including the father can be used for this purpose.

The baby can be put to breast if strong enough to suck; but every effort should be made to observe good hygiene and get the baby to a specialist centre as quickly as possible.

The usual information that babies born at certain gestations ages (7months) do not survive is not correct. Many factors determine the survival of premature babies especially their condition at birth, birth weight and access to centres that can handle them.

Premature babies gain weight rapidly when properly handled. They are usually nursed inside incubators that keep them warm.

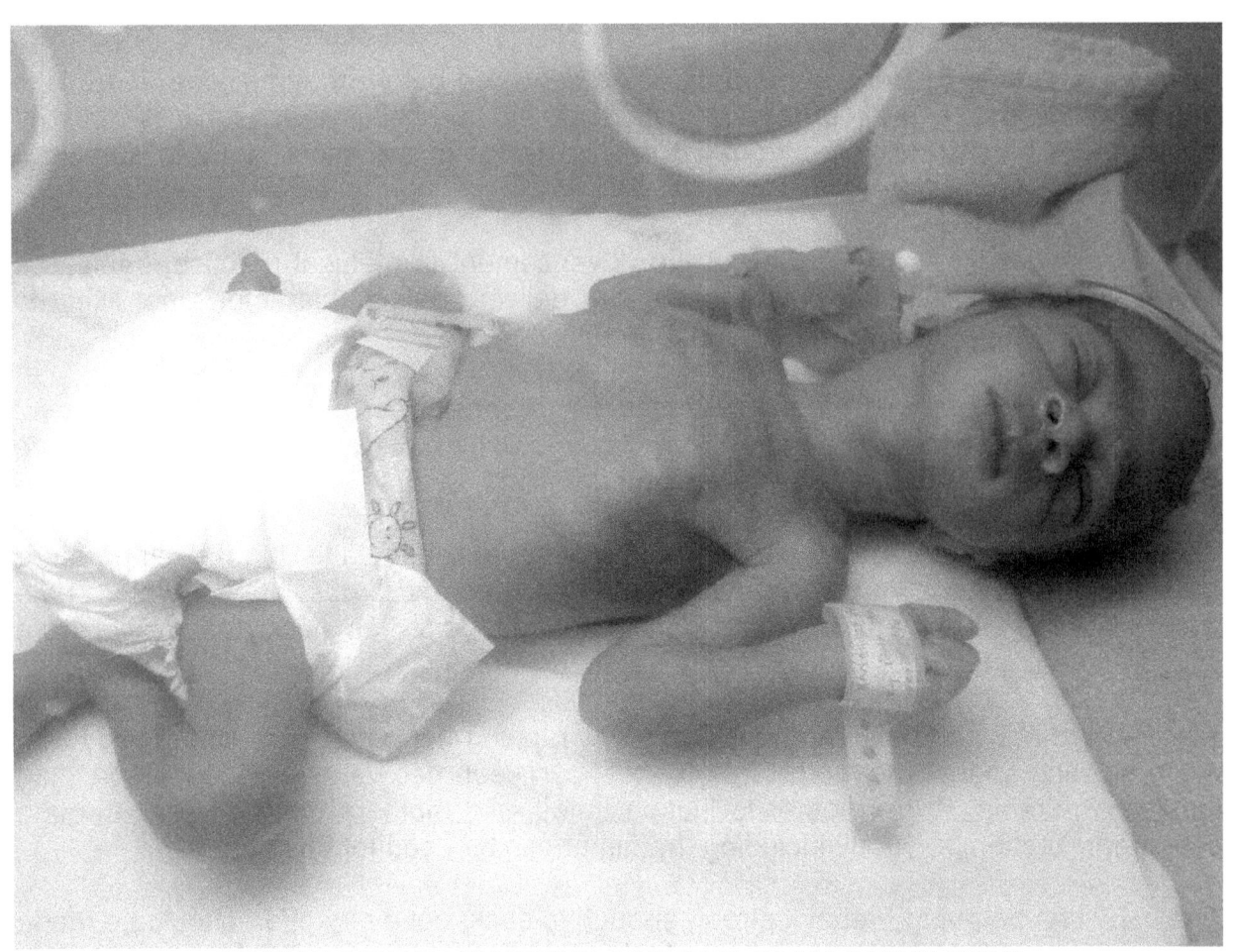

PREMATURE BABY BEING NURSED IN AN INCUBATOR

41

MULTIPLE PREGNANCIES

Twin pregnancies are common in our environment while triplet and quadruplet pregnancies are less common. The babies have their own peculiar problems and they should be addressed individually.

Multiple pregnancies are prone to low birth weight and prematurity because of the limited space in-utero for the development of the babies.

The premature multiple gestations should be handled as already described for the premature babies above. Low birth weight multiple gestation babies should do better than premature babies of the same weight but still need special care like the premature babies. They may have had problems during delivery and therefore need expert care. The second twin usually has more problems than the second twin because of a longer period of labour especially when both babies shared one placenta while in the womb.

Some mothers are usually reluctant when their doctor insists on delivering the babies by caesarean section. This is usually safer for the babies and the mother since it saves both parties the stress of labour and results in usually healthier babies and safer delivery for the mother.

Feeding of the babies should be with breast milk but because the babies are multiple, the mothers assume they should start on artificial feeds immediately after birth. This is not necessarily so. Although the breast feeding of twins and triplets can be stressful, some mothers have practiced exclusive breastfeeding for this category of babies for up to six months. Mothers should seek medical advice on the feeding of these babies.

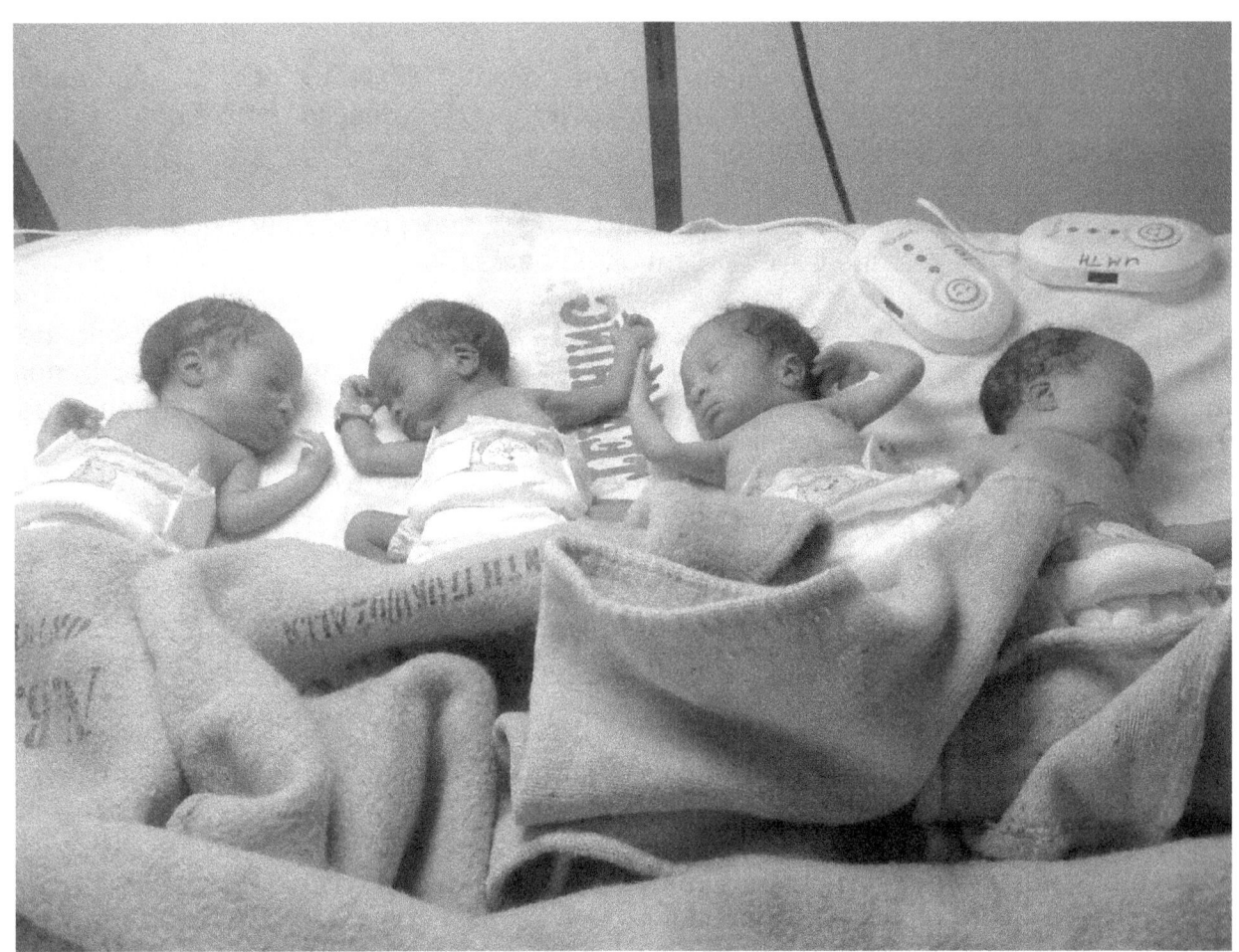

QUADRUPLETS

42

THE SICK INFANT

The sick infant is a source of stress to the whole family and should be handled with care. However, because of traditional beliefs, ignorance and poverty many of these babies arrive in the hospital either in very poor state or too late.

Babies should ideally be taken to see a doctor as soon as they are noticed to be ill or are not behaving the way they used to before. Some of the early signs of ill health in a baby include:

- Fever
- Poor feeding or loss of appetite
- Vomiting
- Excessive crying
- Diarrhoea
- Reduced or poor activity
- Cough
- Poor sleeping
- Abdominal gripes or distension
- Fast or laboured breathing

Please, kindly post a review on this book here.

The author Dr. Gilbert Adimora is a Consultant Paediatrician with the University of Nigeria Teaching Hospital, Enugu and Senior Lecturer in the department of paediatrics, college of medicine, University of Nigeria Nsukka, Nigeria.

E-mail: gilbertadimora@yahoo.com

Website: authorsden.com/gilbertadimora

Tel: 234-8033257771

Fecebook: Gilber Adimora

He is also the author of the books:

The Living water
Healing still the children's bread
The new creature
And others